ROUTLEDGE LIBRARY EDITIONS:
NURSE EDUCATION AND
NURSING CARE

Volume 10

THE NURSING CURRICULUM

THE NURSING CURRICULUM

Theory and Practice

FRED GREAVES

Routledge
Taylor & Francis Group

LONDON AND NEW YORK

First published in 1987 by Croom Helm Ltd.

This edition first published in 2026
by Routledge
4 Park Square, Milton Park, Abingdon, Oxon OX14 4RN

and by Routledge
605 Third Avenue, New York, NY 10158

Routledge is an imprint of the Taylor & Francis Group, an informa business

British Library Cataloguing in Publication Data
A catalogue record for this book is available from the British Library

ISBN: 978-1-041-11658-5 (Set)
ISBN: 978-1-041-11246-4 (Volume 10) (hbk)
ISBN: 978-1-041-11248-8 (Volume 10) (pbk)
ISBN: 978-1-003-65902-0 (Volume 10) (ebk)

DOI: 10.4324/9781003659020

Publisher's Note
The publisher has gone to great lengths to ensure the quality of this reprint but points out that some imperfections in the original copies may be apparent.

Disclaimer
The publisher has made every effort to trace copyright holders and would welcome correspondence from those they have been unable to trace.

The Nursing Curriculum:
Theory and Practice

FRED GREAVES

CROOM HELM
London • New York • Sydney

© 1987 Fred Greaves
Croom Helm Ltd, Provident House, Burrell Row,
Beckenham, Kent BR3 1AT

Croom Helm Australia, 44–50 Waterloo Road,
North Ryde, 2113, New South Wales

Published in the USA by
Croom Helm
in association with Methuen, Inc.
29 West 35th Street
New York, NY 10001

British Library Cataloguing in Publication Data

Greaves, Fred
    The nursing curriculum: theory and practice.
    1. Nursing—Study and teaching
    2. Curriculum planning
    I. Title
    601.73'07'11   RT73
    ISBN 0-7099-3871-3

Library of Congress Cataloging in Publication Data

ISBN 0-7099-3871-3

Phototypeset by Sunrise Setting, Torquay, Devon

Printed and bound in Great Britain by
Biddles Ltd, Guildford and King's Lynn

Contents

Figures and Tables

Figures

Tables

To Rosemary, my wife, always an inspiration. To 'Amy', who helped with the processing, always a challenge. For my students, past, present and future, and to all practising nurses who seek to educate.

Preface

My first book on curriculum (Greaves 1984) presented an overview and analysis of curriculum thinking for nurse education, and a possible model for application to nursing educational practice. This second volume seeks to expand my original broad analysis of curriculum theory and practice which was originally confined to one chapter, and to give a more detailed theoretical account and some general guidance for application to educational practice. The main aim, as well as extending the theoretical discussion, is to present an analytical explanation of approaches to curriculum design, development, and evaluation. This volume also addresses the practical difficulties of building and implementing an effective curriculum for nursing education, and discusses ways and means by which the facilitation of planning strategies can be developed.

The basic approach is through my original thinking concerning the use of the curriculum process as a conceptual framework for dealing with the intentions and purpose, content to be developed, methods to be used, and evaluation approaches which are appropriate for nursing education. There will also be included an account of innovation and change, its implementation and consequences for the nursing curriculum and design teams involved in course development. Within the four main areas of the curriculum process discussed, the analyses developed inevitably deal with some of the important philosophical issues which are of concern for nurse education and the emerging curriculum. The focus here will be on such essential concepts as knowledge, theory and practice, education and training, professional and occupational preparation, teaching and learning as they relate to the development of the nursing curriculum.

Chapter One deals with the concept of curriculum, presenting a general conceptual analysis and comparison of some of the established theoretical views of the early theorists. The component parts of a curriculum and their relationship to each other are outlined as part of the curriculum process.

Chapter Two seeks to question the intentions and purposes of a nursing curriculum and considers the aims and objectives by which the nursing curriculum might secure its aims. There is also an attempt to justify the use of aims and objectives and an account of the theoretical positions and practical usefulness of an objectives approach to course design.

Chapter Three deals with the content of the curriculum and is concerned with its identification, selection and choice. The idea of a core curriculum, its characteristics, applications and organisational frameworks are also reviewed. Knowledge, theory and practice and the use of knowledge in the nursing curriculum are analysed, and attempts are made to show through worked examples of themes and sub-themes, how the content could be developed for nursing courses.

Chapter Four addresses the important issues of curriculum unity and integration and attempts to present a planning focus to unify the curriculum as a whole. There is also a review of some of the theory on integration and some worked examples are presented.

Chapter Five focuses on the selection and use of teaching and learning methods and how these relate to the content and objectives of the curriculum. The distinction between methods and materials is analysed and outline principles are given for designing and selecting learning experiences and the use of curriculum materials. The importance of cognitive and problem-solving approaches are developed and the question of skills in nursing is addressed. This chapter also includes an account of the use and application of teaching and learning in the clinical setting.

In Chapter Six the theme is evaluation and its application to nursing courses. In this theme the measurement, quality and effectiveness of a curriculum are considered, and also whether it works in practice. The main areas of concern are value, judgement, types of evaluation, the significant current theory, and suggested alternative approaches. There is also an attempt to produce some worked examples of evaluation methods.

In the final chapter innovation, change, and their implementation in the nursing curriculum are developed. Attitudes and barriers to implementation are considered along with suggested approaches to increase the facilitation of change and new ideas.

A glossary of important curriculum terms is also included which it is hoped will be of value to those involved in planning teams, development and evaluation groups, or as an aid to those who are making a serious study of curriculum in nursing education.

It is hoped that this book will be of use to all practising nurse teachers, student nurse teachers, and to all nurses involved in the development, operation, and evaluation of the nursing curriculum. This would also include practising clinical nurses and nurse managers at all levels of involvement in the preparation of nurses for their occupational and professional roles.

1

The Concept of the Curriculum

Curriculum is a term much used in education, often without clear understanding of its meaning. Even experienced teachers and other educationalists involved in course design and development use the word in many different situations to mean many different things. The word is incorrectly used to mean anything from a timetable of a teaching programme to an outline syllabus of a course or sometimes the blocks of subjects that are taught in an educational institution. Such common usage is both confusing and generally of little use to those who wish to make a serious study of curriculum and apply correctly its theoretical possibilities to educational practice.

There are many definitions of curriculum available and although there is no general agreement about which serves the most useful purpose as far as education is concerned, each does present a carefully considered view and a set of assumptions that are important for organised education and training. The definitions available are usually in the form of extended conceptual analyses and some may be influenced by particular philosophical beliefs, psychological views, political and social ideals and values. Each one however does attempt to contribute something to the overall meaning and are useful starting points in the conceptual analysis of curriculum. Few if any have developed a sufficiently clear and comprehensive meaning and it seems that curriculum designers and those people involved in the development and evaluation of educational programmes select those particular ideas that fit in with the nature of the educational climate that a specific curriculum seeks to serve.

SOME USEFUL CONCEPTUAL VIEWS OF CURRICULUM

Tyler (1950) was one of the most influential of the early curriculum theorists and has arguably developed a considerable and lasting influence on present day thinking about the nature and function of the curriculum. Following well-established American pragmatism his theories reflect very much the need to organise, and the utility of purpose and concern for an end product of quality and practical application. He views curriculum objectively and in terms of its function and clearly includes teaching and learning as integral parts of it. For Tyler (1950, p1) the function of the curriculum is to set forth the order and scope of what has to be taught so that the learning may be enhanced. The important considerations as far as Tyler is concerned are objectives, outcomes, order and planning, in some sort of rational and systematic sense.

A similar approach developed by Taba (1962, p14) sees curriculum as a design of educational activities, rationally planned and calculated to do certain things. These are to diagnose needs, formulate objectives, select learning experiences and organise those experiences. They include the determining of what to evaluate and the ways and means of evaluating. In Taba's account a number of important and centrally held concepts are put forward which help considerably in curriculum design, development and evaluation. Her specification is a clearly workable statement of curriculum application which not only identifies the components of the curriculum but also their relationship to each other. From Taba's study it is possible to use principles of organisation and at the same time specify the conditions under which the curriculum will operate. The question then becomes not whether to plan but how to plan in the best possible way. Another theorist Wheeler (1967), a contemporary of Taba and much influenced by her work, has developed a systematic and rational approach to curriculum development and evaluation which is offered as a process (Wheeler, 1967, p31). The process is modelled as five distinctive but interrelated steps or stages, each one influencing the other in a dynamic and on-going fashion. The first stage considers the selection of aims and objectives, the second the selection of learning experiences to achieve them, and the third the selection of content (subject material) through which certain types of experience may be offered. The fourth considers the organisation and integration of learning experiences and content with respect to the teaching and learning, and the fifth the evaluation of the effectiveness of all the previous stages. Again the effect is the provision of a set of principles that can be used as a systematic and interactive curriculum instrument. The models evolved from Tyler, Taba and Wheeler have been criticised for their implicit concern with means and ends and their functional emphasis and focus on prescribed learning and specific outcomes. This particular school of curriculum thought has been sometimes unfairly labelled 'the objectives school', and has been thought to be over-influenced by systems theory. Certainly there is a concern with intentions and purpose and clearly there is concern with a systematic approach to curriculum design and evaluation, but surely these are important aspects of educational programmes and provided they are handled with a flexible and sensitive approach they will help in the planning, development and evaluation of the curriculum.

It is important that a distinction is made between systematic approaches and systems in relationship to these particular models. A systematic approach implies a rational and ordered logic to the curriculum whereas systems are concerned with approaches devised from systems theory, and values tightly organised processes with specific inputs and outputs and procedures with feed-back controls. Approaches to curriculum design and evaluation can follow the general systematic models based on objectives, content, method, and evaluation, without necessarily adopting a pure systems approach. The Tyler, Taba and Wheeler models fall within this category and appear to have considerable merit for use with professional and vocational programmes such as nursing and health care courses.

THE INFLUENCES OF JOHN KERR

Kerr (1968) takes an inductive approach to the idea of curriculum and proposes a model that takes a synoptic view of the curriculum from observable data. The focus developed by Kerr is a holistic one and his view of curriculum concerns all of the learning which is planned and guided by the school, whether it is carried on in groups, or individually inside or outside the school.

Kerr's model addresses the sum total of all learning experiences both in the school and beyond the institutional boundaries to wherever the learning is likely to take place, and the range of influence is significantly wider and more profound. The model allows the making of important assumptions about curriculum development, leading to prescriptions for design and evaluation. The conceptual framework guides curriculum choices. The Tyler view of objectives is adopted within the model and is considered as changes in student behaviour which learning is intended to bring about. Kerr identifies four interrelated components of the curriculum as (1) curriculum objectives, (2) knowledge, (3) learning experiences, and (4) curriculum evaluation. The Kerr model addresses certain important questions. They are: what is the purpose of the curriculum? Which knowledge, attitudes, beliefs, and skills are to be valued and used? What learning experiences and methods are to be applied? How are the results to be assessed and evaluated? The answer to these questions can certainly be aided by using the components of the model as areas of focus for the guiding of possible choices in the selection of objectives, content, methods, and evaluation procedures, and their subsequent analysis for inclusion in the curriculum. A criticism of this inductive approach is that one can develop a curriculum that resembles a jigsaw puzzle rather than a continuously evolving system, and for this reason is an unsatisfactory concept of curriculum. Kerr's approach appears to offer for the nursing curriculum a useful set of guiding principles which could be adopted in some relationship with the objectives approach of Tyler and Taba and within the process application of Wheeler. Each have a major contribution to make and an eclectic application will be expanded in this study allowing the development of a curriculum process model for nursing education.

THE COMPONENTS OF THE CURRICULUM

From the conceptual views of the curriculum so far discussed it can be clearly seen that the idea of curriculum relates to educational activities in some sort of rational and ordered way. It has concern for purpose and some sort of clear intent with respect to learning valued knowledge and particular skills using certain learning and teaching approaches and being able to assess the results of its effectiveness. I would suggest the following components as the central concern of the curriculum for nursing education.

(1) The intentions and purposes of the nursing curriculum
(2) The content of the nursing curriculum
(3) The methods of the nursing curriculum
(4) The evaluation of the nursing curriculum

and with the following justification for their use as the main structural and functional frame.

Intentions and purposes of the curriculum

This component is concerned with broad philosophical issues which relate to the fundamental beliefs and values of both nursing as an occupational activity and as a professional area of practice. It also attempts to identify the most appropriate ways to bring these things about, either through training and/or education. From an initial philosophical analysis it is possible to identify the aims and objectives of the nursing curriculum. From such an analysis it is also possible to make a series of decisions based on the available evidence about the nature of nursing and also the views that teachers and others hold regarding the occupational and professional preparation of nurses. The different types of skills and the roles that the nurse will develop are considered as part of the end product and the intended outcomes of the curriculum. Thus an analysis of the role and function of the nurse is necessary together with the appropriate broad areas of knowledge needed to equip her for these.

Content of the curriculum

The term content is used to indicate the knowledge areas of the curriculum and it is necessary to view knowledge as both the theory and the practice of nursing. Both are equal elements of knowledge and this is particularly important for a practical occupation such as nursing. Theory and practice stand in close relationship to each other and a full analysis of this relationship will be given later in this book. For the moment it will suffice to define knowledge for nursing as those subject areas which are fundamental requirements for helping the nurse to learn the practice of nursing in a meaningful way. The content also includes those attitudes, beliefs, and values that are considered proper and desirable for nurses to acquire and which enable them to carry out their occupational and professional activities. The broad skills that nurses need to develop are also included in the content and may be represented initially as the physical or psycho-motor skills, the affective skills or skills of feeling, the cognitive skills or skills of thought and language, the behavioural skills or the interpersonal and communication skills, the social skills, and the technical skills distinctive to nursing. The different skills, knowledge, attitudes, beliefs and values are all within the content, interrelated and integrated to produce a curriculum that is a complete and unified whole and fully representative of the world of nursing. The content must have occupational and professional relevance and be educationally credible and worthwhile.

Methods of the curriculum

The method component of the curriculum is concerned with the methods used to bring about the necessary learning in the students. It includes the selection and arrangement of learning opportunities and the design and use of both teaching and learning strategies which are required to facilitate learning. It also includes the materials used to enable learning and the relationship of the actual methods to the knowledge and skills which we wish the students to learn. The different ways in which knowledge can be presented and the consideration of particular learning theories and teaching style are all important elements of the methods component.

Evaluation of the curriculum

The evaluation component of the curriculum is concerned with the making of value judgements about the effectiveness and quality of its design, development and operation. Whether the curriculum works in practice and whether the intentions and purposes are achieved are integral issues in the evaluation. The quality of educational experience which the students receive and the success of the training procedures built into the programme of study are carefully monitored over the development period of the curriculum and its implementation and continuous operation. The monitoring procedures may be continuous and where they are, they are referred to as formative or on-going evaluations. The evaluation is not just directed at student progress although this is a central part of it, but also at the value and effectiveness of the learning interactions between the students and teachers and the materials that are produced for these interactions.

Determining whether aims and objectives have been achieved and ensuring that the curriculum is being implemented in the appropriate manner are significant aspects of the evaluation. Where the evaluation procedures are directed at specific end-on activities such as the end of a course unit, module, or term of work, or even the end of the course itself, the form of evaluation is called summative. In evaluating the curriculum the usual practice is to include both these general approaches in such a way that as much relevant information as possible is obtained, a comprehensive set of judgements is made and the necessary decisions taken which will continually improve the curriculum. In reality few courses are right the first time and it is part of the nature of developing curricula to make continuing changes and adjustments in the light of evaluation findings. In this way the curriculum is continually developing and the decisions taken through evaluation are part of the shaping and moulding that goes on to enable it to reach a level of excellence.

The four components as a process

The four components of the curriculum briefly described so far have been viewed as discrete elements progressing from intention and purpose to content, to method, and finally, to evaluation. This linear format (see Figure 1) is generally adopted as a set of planning stages in the design of new curricula or the revision of old.

In reality the curriculum tends to be a much more dynamic

Figure 1: The linear format of the curriculum process

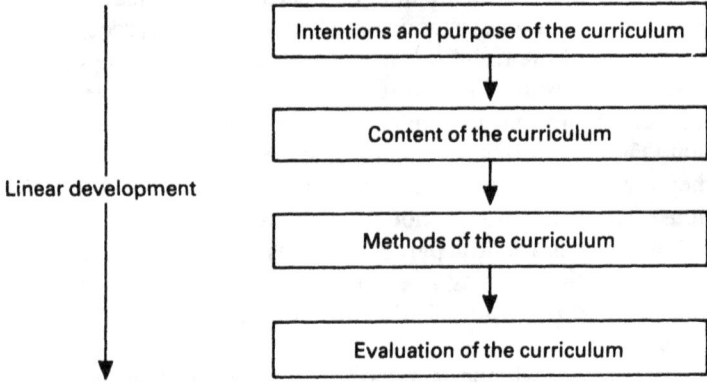

Intentions and purpose of the curriculum
Content of the curriculum
Methods of the curriculum
Evaluation of the curriculum

Linear development

affair with all the components interacting at variable points in its development and in its day to day operation. This dynamic phenomenon of the interacting components of the curriculum (see Figure 2) is often referred to as the curriculum process and is well described by Wheeler (1967, p31) in his study.

The curriculum process seems to be the most useful of the general conceptual approaches to curriculum work in nursing education. It is uncomplicated and free from complex theory with its clear and easily understood components, and offers planners and designers a simple rational approach which has a greater likelihood of being effectively used.

Figure 2: The interacting components of the curriculum process

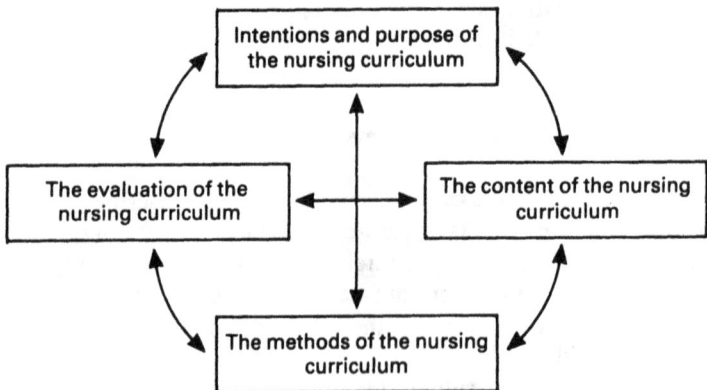

Intentions and purpose of the nursing curriculum
The evaluation of the nursing curriculum
The content of the nursing curriculum
The methods of the nursing curriculum

2

The Intentions and Purposes of the Curriculum in Nursing

The intentions and purposes of the curriculum is the initial focus and the cardinal concern of the first stage of the curriculum process. This primary component allows us to address those important philosophical issues concerning nursing and nurse education which are logically the prerequisite to any decisions about aims and goals. Before a curriculum can be developed, a series of decisions usually has to be taken which indicates the beliefs and centrally held values of those people who will be involved. For nurse educators this means beliefs and values held about the nature of nursing and the occupational and professional preparation of nurses. The decisions which will be made about the intentions and purposes of the nursing curriculum should be based on the evidence available about the nature of nursing. This would include the opinion of authoritative nursing experts, and nursing practice where there is consensus of agreement about the general nature of that practice. There is also clearly a need at this stage to reach some agreement about which fields of knowledge are appropriate and necessary for inclusion in the curriculum, and what are felt to be the educational and training needs of nurses. Questions need to be asked that are directly addressed to the intent of the curriculum and its purpose. It is useful at this stage to consider the intentions of the curriculum as those things which need to be done, and the purpose of the curriculum as the reasons or justifications for doing them. For example:

(a) What is the intention of the design team and what will be the ultimate purposes of the expected curriculum?

(b) What does the school of nursing seek to achieve and how can its intentions and purposes be developed?

The intentions and purposes of the nursing curriculum should be rich in educational significance and as such should be attempting to produce a meaningful and creative curriculum which demonstrates educational credibility and value.

Standing in close relationship to the educational requirements are the occupational and professional requirements. These are no less important and there must be a clear set of agreed intentions and purpose about the nature of the various roles and functions involved and the best way to achieve these. There is a clear need to develop the most appropriate means to these important preconceived results of the curriculum. Careful consideration will have to be given to the actual identification of the general aims of the enterprise and a clear specification of the main goals. This means identifying what the students will be expected to learn and requires the establishment of specific and workable objectives from which the right learning experiences can be developed. At this stage there is also a need to indicate the most appropriate sequence of aims and objectives to what in general terms can be most usefully learned at different stages and levels in the curriculum. Early thinking should also be concerned with the nature of the teaching and learning styles likely to be applied and the general educational climate appropriate for adult students to learn nursing in.

AIMS OF THE CURRICULUM

It is important to be clear about the aims of the curriculum which are internal to education, that is, to be clear about what those engaged in nursing education are trying to achieve.

The word 'aim' is generally used in the curriculum to indicate purpose and intention. Aims are generally developed as an initial broad framework of what the purpose is and what the intentions are. What is the curriculum seeking to do and why is it seeking to do these things? They tend to be based on idealised thinking or grand ideas that are often conventional and include the centrally held values and beliefs of the institution or the occupational group or profession involved. This is certainly the case in vocational and professional curricula such as those used for nursing education. In nursing education the general aim may be to produce a nursing practitioner who fulfills certain expected criteria such as competence, excellence, high standards, professional accountability, and so forth. Such aims are of course highly commendable and desirable, and they often prescribe or recommend something which is worthwile. As such, aims frequently attempt to set out certain fundamental and agreed principles or desirable beliefs and values which nurses hold, or should hold, in esteem.

Aims are vitally important general indicators of the broad issues of concern which form an essential synoptic view of the curriculum and allow important philosophical analyses to be made. For instance, does the institution developing a particular curriculum for nursing have an agreed view of nursing itself, its nature and general role in society? Is there any consensus of opinion on whether the product of the courses should be a generic nurse or specialist nurse? Should all nurses initially be prepared as nurses in the same way in which all doctors are initially prepared as doctors with specialisation following after a common basic training? These are fundamentally important questions for curriculum design and development teams and this form of thinking must logically precede any grand plan.

It is also necessary for questions of this type to address the roles that nurses will be expected to play in their occupational and professional activities as future practising nurses. It is essential that from the very start there are clear and unambiguous statements of intent about the curriculum concerning the various roles that nurses will play. A concerted attempt at role analysis is required so that at least some fairly precise ideas of the nature of the end product are agreed. Although to some extent the aims are directed towards some ultimate target or end product such as the trained nurse of a particular quality, there is also a need to consider the means by which such targets are attained. The idea of means relates to the ways in which these targets are achieved and this in itself raises further questions about the nature of the curriculum to be used. Should the curriculum for nursing be merely a means to a particular set of ends (i.e. the production of the nurse), or should it seek to produce that nurse in a quite distinctive way? To what extent do we want the preparation of the nurse to be an educational experience as well as a professional training? This is an important question that needs to be asked and analysed because it makes a number of quite distinctive demands on the curriculum and on those who will be involved.

The training–education relationship is an important one and the extent to which we are seeking to include them both needs to be clearly implicit within the general aims of the curriculum. The nurse has to acquire the formal skills of the clinical practitioner in the vocational sense of the trained professional nurse. The emphasis of the training is on the dimensions of nursing which set out to produce the expertise of the practitioner and includes, along with the various skills, the nurse's perceptions of the job in the context of commitment and service. During her preparation for nursing the nurse also requires an educational experience that continues to develop her as an individual. This means that the curriculum should among other things help the student to develop a growing awareness of the moral, social, economic, political, and aesthetic dimensions of her work which sets out not only to produce technical expertise as simply a product of 'training', but sets out to show the learner how her skills fit into a wider cultural context. The essence of professional nursing preparation should be experiences that are not productive from training and education diametrically opposed, but as complementary elements that are inter-supporting. Lawson (1979) reminds us that we can talk of trained historians, classicists and mathematicians, yet that training is received within a broad educational experience.

Hardley and Lee (1970) have indicated popular assumptions that training is associated with low status occupations and trades, and education with courses accentuating academic content and high status. It may be a realistic assumption in some areas of general education that training and education do not form part of the same ideological mechanism, but any assumption that education is unrelated to training is clearly an absurd one. Knowledge in all its forms includes elements which are both practical and theoretical and provided they include a cognitive perspective as a fundamental part, then they are part of the educational experience. The level of intellectual difficulty within the curriculum can be just as great in some elements of knowledge that are deemed as training rather than educational, the difference being that these elements are highly specific rather than narrow and constraining. In considering the broad intentions and purposes of the nursing curriculum, they should seek to develop a nurse's skills through programmes that value the intellectual and the cognitive abilities which will enable them to use rational thought, to analyse and to make clinical judgements. Value for intellectual skills should not just relate to the educational parts of the course but to the training elements as well, and the high status normally accorded to academic work is equally important for the more formalised practical aspects of training.

OBJECTIVES IN THE CURRICULUM

In order to achieve the broader aims of the curriculum, which as we have seen involve many philosophical issues, it is necessary to seek some way through which the intentions and purposes are more specific. The objectives are generally speaking the mechanisms through which the aims are achieved. They are more explicit than aims, and as general statements of intent are used to focus more on the actual activities of the students and teachers and often form distinctive strategies to follow. There are many types of objectives and the nature of each is dependent on the precise reason for using each category. The following are examples of objectives:

   (1) behavioural objective,
   (2) teaching objective,
   (3) learning objective,
   (4) performance objective,
   (5) expressive objective,
   (6) educational objective,
   (7) programme objective,
   (8) curriculum objective,
   (9) unit objective,
 (10) module objective.

The above objectives are all attempts to be specific and the word objective is linked to some particular aspect of the curriculum whereby the general aims can be applied more precisely in a distinct context. The behavioural objective is used to state the expected behaviour of a student at the end of a particular piece of learning. It usually involves a set of criteria and a specification of the conditions under which the learning will take place. It may also include some indication of resources or equipment that the student might need to use in order to achieve the objective. There is a general assumption that with the behavioural objective it is possible actually to measure the learning that is to take place. In essence the behaviour of the student is prescribed before the actual learning takes place, so that both student and teacher know what is expected. This form of objective is one of the most widely used in current nursing courses both for classroom work and practical work in the clinical settings. Although influenced by behavioural psychologists of the 'behavioural school', the intentions of educators who use objectives is not to shape behaviour in a particular way as in behaviour modification, but to give a precise statement of intention to the learner that can be measured in some way by the teacher or in some instances by the learner.

The term 'learning objective' is used in a slightly less specific way and really implies a general learning intention which is specified as a statement. The term 'teaching objective' implies an objective statement for the teacher rather than specifically for the student. It usually forms part of the teacher's actual teaching programme or an individual lesson plan. It is much less amenable to measurement. It is more fruitful for both students and teachers to follow the behavioural or learning type objective. When the term performance objective is used the emphasis is on the actual performance of the student. Mager (1962) adopts this approach and points out that to say the student should be able to solve problems would be hardly adequate and asks for a clarification of the conditions under which the actual performance occurs. Expressive objectives relate more to a general expression of intent and tend on the whole to be more flexible and less prescriptive than behavioural objectives. Educational objectives relate to the idea of the planned outcome of education and are generally speaking more akin to general aims. Programme, curriculum, unit, module, and project objectives are all similar attempts to produce objective statements that say what you want the student to be able to do at the end of each. They are all attempts to be specific about intentions and purposes in the curriculum and they have made it possible to be clear in the design of courses with rational planning which seeks to realise in practice the actual aims that have been set in theory.

Any system of curriculum planning may be called rational

when a satisfactory relationship has been developed between ends and means and it is through the use of objectives that this can be achieved. For the present, objectives of a fairly precise form provide a well used method for rational planning in the curriculum. Perhaps the most important thing about objectives for the nursing curriculum is that they should be relevant and meaningful in whichever context they are used. The following is offered as a guide to the characteristics of an adequate objective:

(1) The objective should relate clearly in some way to the educational aim of general nursing.

(2) The objective states what the student will be able to do after the learning experience that she could not do before it.

(3) The objective is developed to a level of detail by specifying the conditions appropriate for the performance.

(4) A standard of performance is clearly stated.

From this it can be seen that objectives are more explicit and tactical in nature than the more general form seen in aims, and they are attempts to describe in the clearest possible terms what is involved in the actual learning and the extent to which the student can or ought to be able to do something at the end of a particular experience. In this sense the expected performance or achievable level of knowledge or attainment of skill is important and requires clear specification. The performance element of an objective sets forth the behaviour to be achieved and is observed as evidence of the learning having taken place. The criteria are clearly required to allow some sort of measure of the desired proficiency or extent of competence to be demonstrated in the students' performance. The objective then ideally describes the behaviour that the student will be demonstrating when the objective is achieved.

Objective statements

The statement of an objective should ideally describe an observable action. A student may be required to state, to construct, to distinguish, to identify, to calculate, etc. The objective statements most likely to be free from ambiguity are those which are open to a lesser number of possible alternative interpretations. The following examples are offered as better key words in objective statements:

(a) to write,
(b) to state,
(c) to identify
(d) to differentiate,
(e) to solve,
(f) to construct,
(g) to list,
(h) to compare,
(i) to contrast.

The following list is of distinctively loaded words which are much to general and vague to be of any real practical use and are almost certain to be interpreted in different ways by different students:

(a) to know,
(b) to understand,
(c) to appreciate,
(d) to comprehend,
(e) to grasp the significance of,
(f) to believe,
(g) to be aware.

The following list is of the expressive type of objective and is useful to indicate an expressed learning intention, (Eisner 1969); an expressive objective does not specify the behaviour the student is to acquire after one or more learning experiences. It does however describe an educational encounter or a situation in which the students are to work, a problem with which they are to cope, or a task they are to learn, but it does not specify what they are to learn from such encounters.

An expressive objective tends to be evocative rather than prescriptive and as such offers the teacher and the student an invitation to explore or focus on issues that are of interest or importance to the enquirer:

(a) to interpret the meaning of patient assessment,
(b) to examine and appraise the effects of anxiety,
(c) to analyse the concept of pain,
(d) to evaluate the responses of the patient,

(e) to critically review the arrangements for,
(f) to visit *x* department and discuss its nature,
(g) to assess the interpersonal responses.

Specific behavioural objectives and expressive objectives can both be usefully incorporated into the nursing curriculum and often are. It is important however that the differences between the two are clearly seen, because the immediate outcomes for the two types can be quite different and they both require different kinds of curriculum activities and evaluation procedures. Behavioural objectives emphasise the acquisition of the known while expressive objectives emphasise the elaboration, modification, and sometimes the production of the new.

THE CLASSICAL TAXONOMY OF EDUCATIONAL OBJECTIVES

The importance of objectives in curriculum design has been advocated for many years (see Bobbitt (1924), Charter and Waples (1929), Dale (1967), Tyler (1950), and Mager (1962)), and these advocates have all insisted that specific and implicit implications within their usage would be helpful to both teachers and learners in their day to day activities. Amongst this new wave of rational curriculum theorists the work of Bloom (1956), and Bloom, Krathwohl and Masia (1964), provided the first classification of objectives in the now classical taxonomy. This set forth a design classification for the intended outcome of the educational process. The cognitive, affective, and later the psychomotor domains (Harrow, 1972) are essentially directed at the intended behaviour of students and stress the relationship of objectives to content, organisation and evaluation. The work of Bloom and his co-workers and the significant contribution of Mager provided a theoretical framework for objective approaches to curriculum design which has been used to some purpose in the design of nursing courses. The critical dimension of a taxonomic system, like behavioural objectives themselves, has been in its potential for facilitating communication in matters of educational planning. There is a need for a standard terminology applicable to learning responses that teachers can evaluate, Krathwohl (1964) identifies four values to a taxonomy:
(1) The actual sharing in the process of classifying objectives

which would help teachers to clarify and tighten the language of educational objectives.

(2) The classification scheme provides a guiding system for describing and ordering the evaluation techniques.

(3) The scheme provides a means of comparative study of educational programmes.

(4) Principles of classifying educational outcomes could produce order among outcomes.

Although the taxonomy is produced as part of curriculum development in general education, it could be made to have significant application for nursing. Although it does not necessarily appear to have direct application to nursing matters it could help teachers to develop thoughtful and rational objectives that take account of cognitive, affective, and psychomotor elements of nursing skills development. An intelligent and carefully considered use of the taxonomy as a frame of reference for the development of nursing educational objectives would be useful in the determination of the intentions and purposes of the nursing curriculum.

Opposition to behavioural objectives in educational usage

However useful the case for specific objectives would seem there are others in the world of education who without rejecting specific objectives outright do have considerable reservations about their use. This does not seem to be the case for nursing courses, however, where they have been used extensively now for some time both in the USA and in the United Kingdom. The reservations of the opposition are worthy of analysis and a comparison of the disadvantages does sound out a warning to the overlavish and dogmatic use of objectives of highly specific form.

Stenhouse (1970) puts forward several reasons for extreme caution in using objectives and indicates some significant reasons for opposing their use. The content can be placed at risk to falsifying methods to meet objectives. Hirst (1969a) also sees this as reducing education to an instrumental role for similar reasons. It is also true that groups of teachers who claim to have agreed their objectives often demonstrate in practice (in the reality of the learning environment) that such agreement was illusory. The last point is of particular importance because there is a widening gap between classroom theory and clinical practice, and also a widening gap between teaching activity in clinical settings (mainly carried out by clinical teachers and ward sisters) and theoretical activity in the classroom (mainly carried out by nurse tutors). The point of issue here is that individual teachers operating in the individual privacy of the classroom may pursue different outcomes to those of clinical teachers operating in clinical experience areas.

More conventional arguments against behavioural objectives are that they are a time-consuming activity and that by pre-stating anticipated results of learning, restriction is placed on the creativity of teaching and learning. There may well be something in the idea that the precision required for the use of objectives is inconsistent with the nature of nursing practice, which can certainly be complex as human interaction and possibly encourages task and procedure approaches. Perhaps emphasis on the particulars of tasks in a nursing context leads to compartmentalisation of nursing practice with a danger of lower levels of learner behaviour becoming trivialised.

Eisner (1967) has warned us that the dynamic and complex process of teaching and learning yields outcomes far too numerous to be specified in educational terms in advance. The implication here for the curriculum and its design and development is that when teachers plan curriculum guides, their efforts to identify overall educational aims that specify the schools' objectives for specific subject matters, appear more like exercises to be carried out, rather than serious attempts to build tools for curriculum development. The argument here is that despite the general acceptance of the idea of objectives, few teachers ever use them or take them seriously enough to influence their own teaching or their students' learning. This must not happen with the curriculum for nursing. The current developments with objective approaches must be more than simply a paper exercise in curriculum intentions.

The way forward with educational objectives in nursing

There is a need to ask questions which will be critical factors in the implementation of objectives for the preparation of nurses for their occupational and professional roles. How can objectives be realised when such a wide separation continues between theory and practice in the learning experiences of the students? How can objectives put into operation in the clinical settings be achieved in an environment where the students are socialised into commitment to the service needs of the institution? How can objectives be realised when there is inadequate supervision from teachers in the clinical settings in which they are placed for formal learning experiences? To what extent can objectives be achieved in a practice learning environment when students are encouraged to use nursing models and problem-solving approaches and the clinical climate is one of task orientation and traditional nursing ritual? These questions point to some of the persistent and long known problems that the students face in the current rites of passage to state registration.

There are no easy answers to these old and persistent problems, but a change in attitudes is the significant factor to a way forward. Even if the occupational and professional preparation of nurses is moved closer to or within general higher and advanced further education, these problems will not disappear overnight. There will still be a need, perhaps even a greater need, to bridge the dimension of theory and practice. Service agencies and educational agencies must develop genuine collaboration and a focal concentration must be developed by teachers to develop lasting relationships with service agencies. A significant shift towards doing this can be achieved by nurse teachers taking increasingly more clinical responsibility to the extent that it is needed to ensure that the clinical practice of nursing is taught to students of nursing by practitioners of nursing. This is something that all of the learned professions do to a greater or lesser extent. As for objectives themselves, they can:

(1) Provide a well worked-out method of rational planning in nursing education.

(2) Encourage nurse teachers and others involved in the preparation of students, to think and plan in detailed specific terms.

(3) Provide a rational basis for the evaluation of learning.

(4) Prescribe the choice of teaching and learning means.

(5) Eventually realise in practice the aims set in theory.

(6) Serve as a medium of communication for learners and teachers, and those managing the curriculum.

(7) Provide a basis for individualised learning and distance learning, and the packaging of learning activities.

It is clear that the intentions and purposes of the curriculum are made explicit through the use of aims and objectives and there is sufficient agreement amongst curriculum theorists to indicate that aims and objectives are a necessary stage in course design and development. Without clear intentions and purpose there is no guarantee that the curriculum will develop in any particular way and to any particular set of conclusions and outcome. Nor would there be any likelihood that developers could recognise the point when they have arrived at a final satisfactory development in its design.

3

The Content of the Nursing Curriculum

The content phase of the curriculum process is the specification and design of what has to be learnt. It is concerned with the forms of knowledge, the various skills, attitudes and beliefs to be acquired by the student, and it also relates closely to the value and relevance of the appropriate subject-matter to be included. In the design and specification of the curriculum content four main areas of importance need to be initially identified. These are in order of sequence:

(1) identification of the general areas of knowledge, skills, attitudes and beliefs,
(2) the selection and choice of the general content areas,
(3) the specific knowledge to be learnt and skills to be acquired,
(4) the nature and form of the content and its integration and unity as a whole.

IDENTIFICATION OF THE CONTENT OF THE CURRICULUM

This has to take clear account of the learners' occupational and professional needs and their general educational growth and development. What do the students need to know and what should the students be able to do? The knowledge and skills that the students are to learn must be relevant and sufficiently appropriate to meet and develop the correct professional and occupational roles that will be required of them. At the early stage of content identification there is a need to ask profound questions about precisely what needs to be taught, what is worth including in the curriculum and which resources are available that can be used to create the desired outcomes and required learning experiences. The factor of relevance cannot be over-stressed at this stage; it is a significant point in the identification of content, and while there is an immediate concern to identify subject areas that should make up the content there is also a need to specify what it would be desirable to learn.

The inclusion of specific content for a nursing curriculum should in itself have educational credibility as well as occupational and professional utility. A continuous focus on the value and worth of the content is essential in order to acquire and maintain this educational credibility. Is the content that we are choosing for inclusion valued and worthy of being included in a curriculum which is pre-eminently aimed at the preparation of nurses, and will the selected content be that which helps the student most to be a good nursing practitioner at the end of the course?

SELECTION AND CHOICE OF THE CONTENT OF THE CURRICULUM

This is inevitably in the first instance concerned with value judgements about what to include and the justification for arriving at certain choices in respect of subject matter. It is useful to focus on those things which *must* be included or those things that learners *must* know or the skills that they *must* acquire. It is also desirable that there is a focus on the things the student *should* know or the skills and knowledge that they *should* acquire. Finally there are the things that they *could* know or the skills that they *could* acquire. In effect there is a definite hierarchy of knowledge and skills which requires an order of priority in terms of usefulness and relevance as far as the broad general areas of subject matter are concerned. Inevitably decisions have to be taken based on appropriate informed choices and this requires a set of decision-making procedures for the selection of content and the specification of what has to be learned. Who is to make the selections and what are the alternative choices available? There is a need to involve key people who will be closely concerned with the running of the courses once the design is developed and implemented. A curriculum development team or a development and evaluation group is essential and this body will be closely involved both with the design of the curriculum and its ultimate implementation, organisation and evaluation. The design team is usually headed by a senior nurse educator who may eventually act as the course leader, specialist subject leaders both nursing and non-nursing, senior clinical practising nurses, (i.e. ward sisters), clinical practising nurses, (i.e. staff nurses), an appropriate nurse manager, a nurse educational manager, a curriculum specialist, (from general education or nursing education), and student representatives from the current student body. From time to time it may also be necessary to co-opt other specialist advisers or experts as is required to help with specific problems. Much will depend on the nature of the course and local requirements. The problems of choice with respect to course content are for the planning team to resolve with decisions being based on the informed judgement of the team members taking into account the necessary statutory requirements of nursing, guidance of the statutory bodies of the day, and the current views regarding nursing practice and nursing theory that are held as authoritative and valued views within the profession. There has to be a considerable amount of consensus amongst the team members on the fundamental issues of the nature of the specific nursing content (concepts and models) and the supporting eclectic subject matter (biology, psychology, sociology), and appropriate links made to the aims and objectives.

Major subject inputs to the curriculum are required to specify major expected outcomes particularly with respect to the way in which the knowledge and skills are to be applied to nursing practice. There also has to be a visible relationship between the general broad areas of content and the methods of dealing with them. Which areas of content, and which ways of dealing with them are to be open to teacher interpretation by way of distinctive forms of teaching and learning approaches? Clearly a degree of flexibility is required about the methods to be used and their precise relationship to the content of the curriculum. Many considerations have to be given to the knowledge and skills that will make up the areas of the main parts of the constituent course programmes and the general form of knowledge has to be carefully considered and the appropriate fields of knowledge from which the essential content is to be selected have to be clearly identified.

The core-curriculum

The core-curriculum usually represents the central area of concern for the content and as a concept itself requires careful analysis, as there is currently considerable confusion about its meaning and practical use. Within curriculum theory the term *core* is used in several different ways and it often means simply the central area of concern within a course or a curriculum, or a particular learning programme. An extreme, but often followed, example of this is all the curriculum areas that are considered compulsory for all the students. It may alternatively represent an area of course patterns which are designed quite distinctively to produce integration to promote more effective learning. The unification of different subject areas may be achieved by developing integration which cuts across subject matter boundaries and this is sometimes achieved through particular learning approaches that consciously seek to bring discrete elements of different subjects together. The concern in these instances is to focus on the students' specific needs and to promote active forms of learning experience that draw subject matter together and to integrate it in the minds of the students. There are clearly differences in the way in which the term 'core' can be used in the curriculum depending on the type of courses being offered and the degree of specialisation and the purpose of particular programmes.

Characteristics of core-curriculum

Certain characteristics are consistently seen that do reflect the design teams' ideas of core. Classically six programmes can be identified that represent different forms of core-curriculum and they can be seen below in order of their deviation from conventional design and organisation.

(1) The core consists of a number of logically organised subjects or fields of knowledge each of which is taught independently.

(2) The core consists of logically organised subjects or fields of knowledge some of which are correlated.

(3) The core consists of broad problems, units of work, or

unifying themes which are chosen because they afford the means of teaching effectively the basic content of certain subjects or fields of knowledge. These subjects or fields retain their individual identity but the content is selected and taught with special reference to a complete unit or to identified themes or problems.

(4) The core consists of a number of subjects or fields of knowledge which are unified or fused in some way. Usually one subject or field serves as the unifying and dominating centre.

(5) The core consists of broad pre-planned problem areas from which there are selected learning experiences in terms of the psychological or social needs and interests of the students.

(6) The core consists of broad units of work or activities planned to promote a greater integration of learning by unifying the subject matter. The method of unification tends to vary from simply a correlation of subject matter around general themes to more complex attempts to deal with problems of learning, the needs of students and the adaptation of the learning environment itself.

Core-curriculum application to nursing courses

With the nursing core-curriculum there is a need to include the distinctive and systematic knowledge of nursing as the core programme and this should centrally dominate in any nursing curriculum. Eclectically derived material taken from such areas as psychology and sociology should be integrated into nursing subjects and related activities rather than simply combined with them. No single field should dominate the core other than nursing itself and where eclectic fields are already in existing programmes there needs to be a refocussing and an orientation into nursing practice. In order to relate the curriculum to the real world of nursing, health care issues in practice, and the immediate needs of the students, the development of knowledge and skills must be taught and learned using problem-solving approaches and must be seen to be integral to the core plan.

Following the philosophical considerations discussed in the previous chapter it should be clear that core-curriculum in nursing requires organisation around a core of nursing ideals, values and beliefs about what nursing is and what nurses do in the practice of their nursing. Clearly the concept of care itself is central to this approach but it needs to be an analysis of care in its distinctive relationship to nursing. So the significant questions for the design of the core-curriculum become which facts, information, concepts, and propositions are relevant to the study of nursing? How is man, society, and health conceptualised by nurses? This form of self-questioning is useful to identify the broad conceptual issues of concern and to develop these as possible leading themes in the core material. At the same time considerable emphasis needs to be placed on the core as the organising centre of the curriculum and the actual structure can be fixed by the broad problems and themes of nursing care and health care issues in society.

Core-curriculum as conceptual and organisational frameworks

In the development of the common core it is necessary for the design team to identify the nature, order, scope and depth of nursing content and set it within a distinctive conceptual framework such as the nursing process or nursing models. These frameworks provide a basic rationale for the selection of learning experiences and also ensure a reasonably positive planning structure for the ordering of knowledge and skills to be learnt within a unified core. The core-curriculum framework can also usefully relate to a wide variety of teaching approaches, learning experiences, and curriculum materials, so that the scope of core units is not just concerned with integrated blocks of subject matter but also with the appropriate selection and organisation of teaching and learning experiences which are design considerations in themselves, and are closely related to the processing of the content.

There are some significant possible difficulties with the use of a core curriculum which can cause problems for curriculum design teams and the ultimate running of the courses and programmes. This is not an attempt to oppose the use of core-curriculum but a warning against insensitive use of the approach and dogmatic expectations. Limitations in the use of core curriculum programmes can be variable and the most common danger is failing to include distinctive and systematic knowledge. This is a particularly pressing problem for nursing as its knowledge is still very much in the process of development. Equally problematic is the marked tendency to combine subjects rather than to integrate them fully. Another common error is to allow one field of knowledge to become dominant over the others: with nursing the subject of nursing should retain its central prominence. Thus, in all attempts to integrate it is the supporting disciplines that need to be applied to the nursing content. Where specialist teachers are being used there is sometimes difficulty in their adapting to broader new fields of knowledge and they are rightly concerned to maintain the rigour of their subject yet at the same time to make the required applications.

Knowledge for nursing: intellectual and utility values

Nursing theory and nursing practice are both integral parts of nursing knowledge and in this respect are the 'knowing' and 'doing' aspects of nursing. They lie together in close relationship and are mutually self-supporting and complementary rather than diametrically opposed.

In the development of the curriculum for nursing there is quite clearly a need for this relationship to be viewed as both inter-related and integrated aspects of nursing knowledge. Because nursing is a practical activity theoretical assumptions about nursing are often regarded with suspicion and it is often believed that there can be no real nursing theories in the sense that the established learned disciplines have theories.

In viewing nursing as a potential knowledge area for the curriculum it is essential that the design team have a clear conception of what knowledge means. The idea that nursing is practical and therefore not theoretical rests on a misconception of what knowledge is. Practical activities are preceded by thought and reason and however simple must take account of theory. Knowing what to do, how to do it, and why it needs to be done are all bound up in the actual performance of nursing, and knowing and doing in that sense belong to the same locus of knowledge which include the theory and practice. For the curriculum in nursing education nursing knowledge cannot be purely practical or in fact purely theoretical in any separate way for both are part of nursing activity and consequently the knowledge of nursing itself.

The word knowledge in general usage refers to some sort of clear and certain mental perception that includes awareness and understanding of something. It usually requires learning to achieve cognisance of facts and information in order for it to be understood. Possession of knowledge in this sense is to 'know' or to be aware and familiar with the possessed knowledge to be learned. Knowledge should not be viewed by nurses as just collections of theories that merely exist to guide their practice. The theories developed by nurses should offer a speculative system based upon the explanation of observed facts or phenomena that ultimately involve the development of laws and principles consistent with knowing what is the case and why in nursing contexts. Certainly nursing knowledge must exhibit its own concepts and the relationship between its concepts, but these must also embrace practice or the performance of nursing in accordance with theory which includes, knowing how and knowing why, and essentially doing nursing care well.

The idea of practice and the practical must be seen as central to nursing knowledge for the concept of practice includes notions about criteria and standards of performance for nursing. To achieve the product of good care the nurse in the practice of nursing has to acquire and use intellectual skills as well as practical skills and for the curriculum there is a necessary distinction and link to be made between them. The significant point is that both sets of skills rest within the same continuum of knowledge. Intelligent purposeful activities such as nursing care depend upon the informed use of both types of skills. For example the nurse planning care for the patient goes through the activity of thinking and this thinking is the preparatory action as she gets ready to implement some element of care. This activity of thinking is strictly speaking using theory or thinking about the practice that has to be done. The nurse is acting cognitively within her mind and subsequent action is based upon her theory as it is used to shape her plan of nursing approaches and care. In this sense the relationship between theory and practice is an interrelationship and the theory and practice are part of the same endeavour.

Knowledge for the curriculum

The problem with nursing knowledge at present for the curriculum can be clearly seen in previous attempts in the past to fragment content into theory and practice. This has occurred in the separation of content to be taught in the classroom and the actual practice to be taught in the practical rooms of the schools of nursing. Similarly the division is extended into a wider dichotomy with an assumption that theory is taught in the school and that practice is taught in the service experience areas of the hospitals. Emphasis has been on learning and practising skills in isolation from the idea of nursing as a whole. Clinical expertise is proportionally theory and practice and each is complementary to the other. In this respect the curriculum should incorporate the relevant applications of knowledge whereby the student can develop the necessary insights and clinical judgements which take account of that knowledge.

The knowledge base should also be used to enhance the nurses' ability to deal with problems by providing the learning experiences that allow for the application of theory into contexts of nursing practice that present the opportunities for the student to engage in actual problem solving.

Developing knowledgeable nurses means more than simply getting nurses to learn information and facts and rests more on the assumption that having knowledge which is worthwhile depends on the holder of the knowledge possessing meaningful understanding of that knowledge and a capacity to apply it in the practice of nursing. The curriculum arrangements need to focus on the development of that capability. The knowledge to be learnt also requires that it be relevant and appropriate for today's nurses and free from the dogmatic traditional constraints of the past. Although we have advanced the development of formal nursing knowledge over recent decades we have not as yet effectively systematised our application of this knowledge into the reality of nursing practice. To apply existing knowledge effectively into the curriculum we need to re-analyse the scope of nursing knowledge and try to agree on how the emerging knowledge can best be used.

These are significant problems for the design and development of the curriculum and the following propositions are offered as a guide for the possible consideration of knowledge as curricular content:

(1) Knowledge of nursing or 'nursing knowledge' should include both theory and practice as inter-supporting elements of the activity of nursing.

(2) Nursing knowledge should include information, concepts, skills, and practices that are relevant, useful and capable of being

known and learned in order to have direct utility value for the practice of nursing.

(3) The knowledge included should be worthwhile and transferrable to the nursing of patients.

(4) The developed knowledge included in the curriculum has to have consensus in the sense that it needs to be agreed and acceptable and wherever possible based on the best available evidence.

(5) The knowledge used in the curriculum should help develop explanations of current practices, encourage critical analysis, influence problem solving, and help establish in the students abilities to develop scientific approaches of enquiry.

(6) The future preparation of nurse practitioners should be based on the use of knowledge through educational experiences that prepare the aspiring nurse for knowledge creation and innovative nursing practice.

In the development of a curriculum for nursing there is quite clearly a need for the relationship of theory and practice to be seen as equal elements of the central content of the curriculum, and no useful purpose can be gained from creating or perpetuating further division between theory and practice. Knowledge cannot realistically be called either practical or theoretical and any discrimination of subject matter into practice and theory when seeking purposeful curriculum organisation is inevitably bound to increase the already existing artificial divisions in the content of the curriculum. Consequently no sharp distinction should be made between the practical and the theoretical and the legitimate exercise for the moment should be for curriculum developers and implementers to seek the most effective arrangements for integrating theory and practice.

Skills to be included in the nursing curriculum

In the past most of the skills set within previous curricula have been mainly of the psychomotor type, the necessary physical skills of nursing the patient. Many of these skills have been developed through traditional practices of the past and are those elements of nursing practice which have been carried out by generations of nurses, passed on by generations of nurses and ritualised into the procedure and policies of the present day nurses.

Although a significant amount of traditional practice involves skills which are time-tested in terms of clinical effectiveness over many years of application to the care of patients, few stand up to fundamental scientific explanation. Their validity and reliability in scientific terms is at best empirical and they are often viewed as lacking in support through tested and verifiable theories. Those within the profession who are in pursuit of scientific explanations of nursing care and a rational set of scientific principles upon which future practice can be based are currently developing a research base from which new and alternative practices can emerge. There are also those who see the traditional practices as time-tested and effective over many generations, and who place considerable emphasis on the ideals which explain nursing in terms of it being an art in the vocational sense, but who accept gradual change in practice as it falls in line with new technology. Clearly the curriculum has to take account of both these positions in the development of the skills area of the content. They do however require quite frequent reviews and as practice is influenced through research, the developed changes in clinical practice will need inclusion in nursing courses.

Nursing of course does not just rely on the physical skills of care though emphasis has been placed there in training nurses in the past. There is an undisputed need to give more space in the curriculum to the development of cognitive skills whereby the thinking, analytic, and problem solving abilities of the nurse are encouraged and the 'thinking' skills and the traditional psychomotor skills are brought closer together and linked to the development of psycho-social abilities such as interpersonal and communication skills. Such behavioural skills are implicit within a wide range of nurse–patient interactions and require a collective application in the curriculum within a wide range of care contexts. A collective skills element is therefore an essential, focal part of the whole.

The shape and form of the curriculum for nursing

An analysis of the desired content needs to be made with respect to the way in which it will be generally structured to produce a grand overall design. This requires a structured organisational pattern that includes both the boundaries and the limitations of a particular curriculum. The organisation should reflect the main organisational pattern through the main concepts and principles of nursing and at the same time develop an effective inter-relationship between the various elements of inter-supporting subject matter and skills. This particular focus will be more fully developed in the next chapter but for the moment there is a need to identify the correct and appropriate level on which subjects should be dealt with, and the desired level of intellectual difficulty and skills competence that will be needed. Any consideration of the content in terms of its design features must also take account of the methods of teaching and the learning experiences to be created. This vital link between content and methods involves important decisions concerning the proposed use of distinctive methodology such as units, modules, themes, sub-themes, and the like. It also relates to the actual instructional approaches to be used and choices to be made regarding the amount of formal or informal learning, self-paced individualised or group-paced collaborative approaches, and the extent to which packaged learning can be used and the form of the curriculum materials to be involved. These all have a strong influence on the actual moulding of the grand design itself.

The nature and distinctiveness of certain subject areas by their innate logical order may well indicate the type of learning approach which is likely to be of most help to the students. Even the sequence of dealing with specific material is often determined by the conceptual structure and principles inherent in the subject itself. Clearly content must relate to the methods to be used to enable the desired learning to take place in any sort of rational order. Equally of concern is the need to link the content to the aims and objectives of the curriculum, and decisions have to be made about the expected outcomes to be achieved. The content in its developed relationship to aims and objectives should not be allowed to become distorted or in fact trivialised in a blind attempt to secure objectives. Distinctive material whether distinctive to nursing or borrowed from other disciplines should be allowed to retain its individual character and rigour. Similarly the subject material selected for inclusion in the content of the curriculum requires relevance in that certain aims and objectives which are currently held as important for nursing courses need to be achieved. A close relationship can be obtained between content and aims and the purpose and intentions of the curriculum can be developed without damaging the excellence of distinctive subject disciplines. With the likelihood of considerable future change in the content of nursing it will be necessary to review frequently the nature of the content for the curriculum of nursing. The content must increasingly be fully representative of the present state of the developments in nursing knowledge research and theoretical advancements. Design, development, and evaluation teams should ensure that the content of the curriculum is directed at the production of a professional nurse practitioner and that the student is given an educational experience as well as an occupational preparation, and that the experience is more than simply a rite of passage to registration as a nurse.

From syllabus to curriculum content

There is considerable difference between the syllabus and the finished curriculum. With most attempts in the past at producing courses for the training of nurses the syllabus was given by the statutory body of the day and it then became the job of the nursing school staff to interpret that syllabus and create a curriculum. This was usually done within very close guidelines and regulations that tended to place almost impossible constraints on the staff and dampened any real curricular creativity. The situation is now of course changing with increasing accountability and responsibility for course design being delegated to the schools themselves.

Where a syllabus is a given one it is usually an outline syllabus and whether a guide is given with it or not it is really no more than a list of subjects to be taught on the course. The list itself may or may not be in any sort of logical order although it does usually present some form of distinctive grouping of subjects. The actual ordering of the subject areas is an early consideration that needs to be done in the planning of the content. Which areas of the content need to be learned first by the students and in what priority of sequence should other areas follow? It is important to remember that some subjects do have an inherent logical development within themselves and that certain topics naturally precede others with respect to ease or difficulty of learning and moving from simple to complex elements. The concept of unity is perhaps important at this stage and that each component of a subject is seen as a complete unit. With such completeness it is then possible to reorder it in the overall sequence of events if the need arises. When an initial proposed order of progression of the subject matter has been established there is a need to expand the content in more detail.

Expanding the content through themes and sub-themes

Themes are planned devices which help in the expansion of the subject matter and in developing its progression in the curriculum. They can also be used to integrate content but their use in integration will be the focus of the next chapter. In this chapter the use of themes will be dealt with in terms of expanding the subject matter. A theme represents a recurring set of events that are developed in a progressive manner as central concepts and main ideas within a subject or across subject boundaries. A sub-theme is a sub-division of a theme where the level of detailed explanation is increased or further expanded. It is usual where an objectives approach is being used in the curriculum for the themes to have integral aims or general objectives related to them and the sub-themes to have fairly specific objectives suggested. Hence in the use of themes in expanding the content a direct attempt is made to link content to intentions and purpose and to develop a progression of the content at the same time.

It might be useful at this stage to consider some examples of how themes and sub-themes could be used and developed. By way of example it is useful to look at a part of a nursing syllabus and to consider a possible format of themes for expanding the subject material and this might be done in the following way. The examples offered are merely an attempt to present the mechanics of dealing with themes and to suggest certain possibilities for the nursing curriculum.

The use of themes

Example one. Subject: the professional development of nursing

Aim. To enable the student to develop insights into the professional development of nursing and analyse the significant historical and social perspectives involved.

Objectives. (1) To identify what is meant by the concepts 'profession' and 'professional nurse'. (2) To examine the extent to which nursing as an occupational group has credible professional identity. (3) To analyse the arguments for regarding nursing as a semi-profession or a profession in evolution. (4) To examine historical and social contexts and trace their influence on the professional growth of nursing. (5) To examine critically the authority and controlling influences in nursing and their effect on professional development.

Theme one: nursing as a profession

The professional nurse and the concept of professionalism including the image and the reality of nursing. The characteristics of a profession and the meaning and nature of professional growth. The dimensions of professionalism and professional evolution in nursing. Nursing as it is perceived by other professional groups. The nature of nursing authority and accountability and responsibility in nursing. Current issues and developments significant for the professional control of nursing.

Sub-theme A: the evolution of professional nursing

Historical perspectives, the origins of nursing in the 18th and 19th centuries.
The influences of Florence Nightingale and early training approaches.
Images and perspectives, values and beliefs of nurses.
Vocational ideals and the Victorian Nursing Ethic.
The nature of nursing practices and influences on their development.
The development and socialisation of nurses into occupational roles.

Sub-theme B: professional control of nursing

The development of public and State recognition.
The establishment of statutory bodies and mechanisms of control.
The evolution and reforming of the statutory bodies.
Legal authority controls and powers in nursing.
Professional, educational, advisory, and evaluatory functions of the professional bodies.

The use of themes

Example two. Subject: the theoretical perspectives of nursing

Aims. To identify the nature of nursing and the emerging conceptual frameworks and models.

Objectives. (1) To explain what is meant by the term nursing. (2) To compare, contrast and analyse the various conceptual accounts of nursing. (3) To consider the possible application of conceptual models to nursing practice. (4) To discuss the extent to which nursing can establish a distinctive body of knowledge which is capable of guiding and supporting clinical practice. (5) To explain the possible relationships between the nursing process and the currently emerging conceptual models of nursing.

Theme one: the concepts of nursing

An analysis of the established concepts of nursing and the current conceptual frameworks for practice. The use of conceptual analysis to gain a perception of the nature of nursing. The need for a systematic frame of reference that can be used to guide nursing practice. The use of established theory from other disciplines and its application to nursing. The pursuit of a distinctive order of nursing knowledge which can be verified and tested in practice.

Sub-theme A: nursing theory and models for nursing practice

Nightingale's perspectives of nursing.
Contributions to nursing theory and models for nursing practice in the work of: Henderson, Abdellah, Roy, Johnson, Roper, King, Orem, Macfarlane and Castledine, Patterson and Zderad.
Systems, interactionist, and developmental models and their application to nursing.

Sub-theme B: nursing knowledge

Typologies of nursing that focus on the biological, behavioural, and social needs of the patient.
Identification of the appropriate parts of the above disciplines basic to nursing, and justifying an eclectic use of this knowledge to support nursing practice.

Defining concepts of care and analysing these concepts for possible application to models of nursing.
Considering objective approaches and systems theory and their application to the individualised care of patients.
Describing the nursing process and analysing its phases for nursing care application.

The use of themes

Example 3. Subject: care

Aims. To identify and analyse the concept of care and consider its characteristics in relationship to nursing.

Objectives. (1) To define and analyse the concept of care and explain its meaning. (2) To consider the characteristics of care through physical, psychological, social, and philosophic perspectives. (3) To explain the meaning of self-care, collaborative-care, and care as a sharing activity. (4) To discuss the meaning and development of institutional care. (5) To describe the possible use of the concepts of caring as a basis for providing nursing care. (6) To compare and contrast health care and nursing care.

Theme one: care as the central focus of nursing

The concept of care, analysis and definitions of meaning. The characteristics of care through philosophic, social, and psychological perspectives. Physical care, practical caring, and spiritual care. Giving and receiving care. Care based on scientific knowledge. Care as enabling, helping, assisting, supporting, motivating, facilitating, and teaching. Care in institutions. Care by individuals and by groups. The aims and goals of caring.

Sub-theme A: health care concepts

Concepts of health care, analysis and definitions of meanings. Comparison of caring and curing. Care as health maintenance and social support. Caring as a coping strategy. Mutual care, care sharing and self care. Health care and nursing care comparisons. The cause and effect of institutional care. Health education as care. Caring practices in health promotion and maintenance. Collaborative health care practice.

Sub-theme B: nursing care concepts

Concepts of nursing care, definitions, analysis and meanings. Using the concepts of care as a basis for nursing. Philosophical, moral, and ethical care in nursing. Physical, social, and psychological care in nursing. Communication and interpersonal skills of caring in nursing. Technical care and caring practices in nursing. The concept of self care and its relationship to nursing. The concept of collaborative care and its relationship to nursing. Nursing care in institutions and in the community. Comparisons of cure and care activities in nursing. The care giving role of the nurse and the care receiving role of the patient. Teaching care, and health educational care in nursing. The nature of care relationships in nursing.

The three examples given above demonstrate how part of a unit of subject material can be developed into themes and sub-themes in order to give some expansion to the content as the syllabus is developed in a vertical progression. Each theme and its related sub-themes are preceded by a general aim and constituent objectives thus establishing the direct link between aims, objectives and the subject area of the content. It is also necessary to extend this vertical progression into the methodology to be used and to include some relationship to evaluation. This relationship then completes the application of the curriculum process to the content and the following examples are offered:

The use of themes

Example 4. The methodology

Sub-theme A: the concepts of nursing

Teaching methods
(1) Four sequenced lectures to establish the framework of the concepts of nursing and the development of conceptual frameworks.
(2) Each lecture followed by the division of the main class into a number of small tutor-led discussion groups to consider material in more depth.
(3) To be followed up during the same week by tutor-led seminars with four students making prepared contributions to the proceedings.

Learner activities

The students will

(1) make a conceptual definition of nursing,
(2) write short notes on the concept of nursing models,
(3) make a search of the literature on the concept of nursing,
(4) broadly compare and contrast systems, interactional and developmental, types of nursing models,
(5) follow the reading assignments suggested in the students' study guide to this sub-theme.

The use of themes

Example 5. The evaluation

Sub-theme A: the concepts of nursing

Evaluation approaches

(1) Analysis of individual student's performances in tutorials and seminars.
(2) Evaluation and discussion of students' written material in their work books.
(3) Discussion of the outcome and problems of the literature search.
(4) Set essay assignment on 'the concept of nursing' and revision of draft schemes with individual students.
(5) Give structured feedback on essays with emphasis on structure, content, text referencing, and bibliography.

4

The Nature of Curriculum Unity and the Integration of the Content of the Nursing Curriculum

In considering the overall and uniform nature of the content as a whole it is necessary to develop a pattern of design which is logical in its scope and follows an appropriate sequence of events and development. The individual subject areas of the content have to be looked at in terms of their interrelationships and the extent to which they can become part of the total picture of the content. The aim of integration is the promotion of the concept of wholeness or unity. The approach to a unification of the subject matter is mainly through the structuring of content into a correct order and sequence using appropriate integration techniques so that the students are assisted in assimilating and integrating knowledge in their own minds. Three basic concepts relate to the unity of curriculum content and they are respectively: (1) the scope of the content; (2) the sequence of the content; (3) the integration of the content.

THE SCOPE

The scope of the content concerns questions about what to include and what to exclude as far as the selection of subject matter is concerned and includes the broad framework of the range and extent of each area to be covered. Determining the scope must include some reference to aims and objectives and the range of learning experiences. Considering what is to be included in the content is sometimes referred to as 'determining the scope' and it can be seen to operate at four levels. First there must be decisions regarding what to include as a whole in the major areas within which the curriculum operates. Should the concern be with certain subjects that are basic to the understanding of human caring such as those within the behavioural sciences and humanities? Should the selection draw from the life sciences in that these may help the nurse understand the physical factors of care? Should material be developed that addresses health care and health education? Is there a need to include a study of the abnormal in terms of pathological considerations that are appropriate for the study of nursing? This sort of questioning is directed at the identification of the subjects which are thought to be eclectically desirable for the underpinning of the base of nursing practice. These have been considered at length before (Greaves, 1984), and viewed as the essential antecedents to distinctive nursing knowledge.

There is a need within the scope of the content to determine which antecedent subjects to include as subjects which are essential bases of nursing and from which elements can be selected to increase the understanding of nursing. These bases have been outlined in a previous volume (Greaves, 1984, pp 53–9) and a supporting justification offered for their inclusion in the curriculum. Similarly there is a need to identify the existing distinctive knowledge of nursing at least to the extent that it has currently been developed, and decisions again have to be made about what to include and what needs to be included.

There is a second level of scope which looks at the area of a distinctive subject and considers what might be borrowed and used. This eclectic use of knowledge draws on and extracts from the particular established discipline concerned without necessarily accepting the total area of ideas and beliefs within the totality of the discipline. A third level of scope determination concerns the individual teachers working from the curriculum at classroom level and involves independent decisions about how much material can be developed within a particular period of time and where the emphasis should be placed within certain subjects and topics. A fourth level of scope relates to individual lessons concerning the areas to be dealt with and the extent they are to be covered and the level of intellectual difficulty involved.

Taba (1962, p382) has suggested that the pattern of the curriculum should adopt a certain idea of scope which focuses on certain centres of organisation. Such centres of organisation can be seen to operate through unitary themes, or modular themes, and these can determine the way in which the content can be mapped out in a curriculum and also be organisers for teaching and learning purposes. Scope therefore, is not just concerned with the content in terms of areas to cover or main ideas to develop, but is also concerned with the variety and form of learning experiences and the appropriate teaching approaches that help to form these learning activities. The way in which they are arranged is important, because the actual teaching–learning interactions can be structured into the main curriculum plan in such a way that they act as powerful potential integrators between content and methods.

In dealing with the scope of the content certain basic principles can be usefully followed and these can also act as a general guide for making decisions:

(1) There is a need to work from basic generalisations or universal thinking about the content, progressively towards specific or particular elements.

(2) The initial decision-making should be concerned with the identification of the major areas of knowledge to be included.

(3) The content to be included must be educationally worthwhile.

(4) The content must be occupationally relevant for nursing.

(5) The content should be professionally relevant for nursing.

(6) The scope must determine the appropriate skills, attitudes, and beliefs which the students need to acquire.

(7) The scope should determine the appropriate intellectual and practical level of difficulty in the content.

(8) The scope needs to take account of whether additional external expertise is needed from outside the field of nursing.

(9) The scope of the content should reflect the necessary educational technology to be included and the curriculum materials to be used.

(10) The scope ought to include consideration of the basic form of assessment and examinations to be used.

Inevitably when the scope of curriculum content is being determined there will be concern for the traditional approaches of the past which may well be thought to have stood the test of time. Certainly the content may have to take account of traditions and the nature of previously developed or currently established curricula in nursing education, but decisions about what to include must be based on objective thinking. In essence the knowledge and practices to be included must rest on decision making that is based on whether the subject matter to be selected is valuable, relevant, and can be justified as worthwhile for a nursing curriculum. A final factor of pragmatic significance for the scope of the curriculum is the external influences that may affect its development. The possible effects of financial implications, availability of resources and staff, the policies of the institutions, statutory and controlling bodies, local and central government departments, may all have a profound influence on the direction and development of the curriculum. These external agencies can mediate and produce scope determinants to which planners are forced to give account. On the other hand external agencies can be sought for expert opinion on particular subject disciplines or subject fields.

THE SEQUENCE

If scope is defined as the main areas to be included in the content of the curriculum and the extent to which emphasis is given to them, sequence can be considered as the order in which the content and its processing is presented to the learner. Sequence is related to the progression and correct development of content and the main aim is the systematic yield of predictable student learning performance. If scope is related to what to include in the content, sequence is related to when to include something. It involves a spatial relationship between the content and its processing and the order of difficulty is often seen as fundamental. In almost any sequence there is a tendency to move from simple to complex elements of the subject matter, and from concrete operations to abstractions, and from the immediate issues of concern to the more wide and remote. In these instances things which are easier to learn are presented before things which are harder to learn. The factor of immediacy is also important and relates to the 'when' criteria, or the point in progression at which the students are ready for a particular element of the content. Similarly there is concern that certain topics or materials should have quite specific value to the students at particular levels in the curriculum. The sequence of design is strongly related to the 'when' criterion and to the question of duration, so that when a topic or subject is introduced the extent to which the students will be exposed to the content is significant. Thus the timing and the length of units or modules is a necessary concern, as is the principle that information and learning experiences presented at the time they are of greatest use to the students.

The logic inherent within various subjects and disciplines is also important for the sequencing of content. Most subjects do have an inherent logic and order which is quite distinctively sequenced, and it would be foolhardy to interfere with the natural order of a subject's material when it is presented for learning purposes. This rational pattern of order means for learning purposes that certain concepts, theories, and topics precede others in the natural enfolding of the material. Taba (1962, p 81) would use the logic of the content to pursue those questions that represent this order of rational pattern. Incremental logic or the incremental presentation of knowledge to the students is considered essential. In line with this rational incremental progression of content is the thinking of Gagné (1965) who would consider the prerequisite knowledge and move from the known to the unknown, from concrete to abstract, and from universals to specifics. Within these approaches there is a step by step logic within the nature of the subject matter and a sequence of progressive presentation that facilitates the student's ability to come to terms with the subject.

Sequencing should finally relate to objectives in the development of the content and the way in which the content is ordered. In order to achieve the aims and objectives of the curriculum and the expected learning outcomes it is important that the learning objectives are sequenced appropriately in the most advantageous order. The point here of course is that the objectives and the content being dealt with must be evolved together in close proximity, and that the correct teaching and learning activities should follow the sequence.

INTEGRATION

Attempts to integrate the content of the curriculum do to a greater or lesser extent follow on from scope and sequence although there is some overlap between the three. A common assumption about integration is that it takes place within the mind of each student and that this internalised integration should be a major aim of the curriculum. From a design and planning point of view it should be seen as a series of operations which attempt to produce balance and unity to the curriculum. From a content point of view this means the production of a functionally complete whole.

The production of this complete whole requires that each subject and discipline included for the nursing curriculum should have a clear relationship to each other and that different elements of different subject areas need to be brought together for presentation into distinct nursing perspectives. For instance, elements of sociology and psychology often have overlapping significance or common similarity, which can usefully be brought together to focus on a specific nursing theme or context.

Welch and Slagle (1980) have stressed the importance of the internalisation of knowledge by the students and have suggested integration as a way of organising the curriculum to assist the students in analysing and applying the concepts and principles of nursing care into nursing practice. With internalisation there is clearly some danger in assuming that students can easily absorb differentiated knowledge and at the same time integrate it into their minds. There is in reality a greater chance of positive internalisation of knowledge within students if the areas of knowledge which we desire them to learn are integrated or at least correlated in some systematic way within the course design. Such structuring can be achieved in a number of ways and the following are some examples:

(1) Common core content.
(2) Broad conceptual frameworks.
(3) Organisational schemes of work.
(4) Problem solving themes.
(5) Projects and assignments.
(6) Resource units.

Common-core and its relationship to integration

Taba (1962, pp 407–12) sees core-curriculum as an ambitious attempt to provide for integration, to serve the needs of the students and to promote active learning. Within this approach she also includes problem-solving techniques and the unification of subject matter correlated around themes or problems. Wheeler (1967, p 259) also has identified core-curriculum as an attempt to integrate by concentration on functions, problems, or situations. Core programmes certainly show some common characteristics which attempt to promote unity of content. For instance there is often an attempt to try to meet the needs common to all of the students who are following a particular course. There is generally an attempt to break down the traditional subject division boundaries that exist between disciplines and in order to do this the core programme combines with other courses or elective options. Where it is sought to integrate core programmes, use is often made of a wide variety of teaching and learning approaches that incorporate enquiry methods or problem solving.

Broad conceptual frameworks

Integration as an approach to the organisation of content in the curriculum can be explained as a direct contrast to programmes with compartmentalised subject areas which have perpetuated a fragmented curriculum. This is well demonstrated in the nursing curriculum of the 1950s and the 1960s when subject areas were clearly seen to be insular and isolated from the general nursing content. Traditional subject barriers can limit dangerously the students' view of the whole picture or confine study to insular areas of knowledge rather than to the central focus of the course which for a nursing curriculum must by definition be nursing. For the nursing content there has to be a clear idea of what it is one wants to integrate and to open up the different supporting subject areas (i.e. physiology, psychology, sociology), so that they can be applied to a whole view of nursing and a whole view of the patient. The use of broad conceptual frameworks can help to achieve the unity which is desirable. The frameworks can deal with different forms of knowledge or categories of knowledge that support the key concepts and basic themes of nursing. Using conceptual frameworks in this way allows the centrally important material to be mapped out as the broad structures of the curriculum. The nursing process can usefully serve as such a mapping scheme and conceptual models of nursing can be used in a similar way. (Greaves, 1984) The following are examples of broad conceptual frameworks (Greaves, 1984, pp 54–8)

(1) The biological basis of nursing practice.
(2) The psychological basis of nursing practice.
(3) The sociological basis of nursing practice.
(4) The anthropological basis of nursing practice.
(5) The pathological basis of nursing practice.

Each of these five perspectives can be arranged as the eclectic framework with integrative links to specific nursing knowledge (see Figure 3). They collectively form the essential antecedents for nursing knowledge when the appropriate selected elements of each are applied to nursing contexts.

Such a framework allows the students to use knowledge from these disciplines to produce biologically, psychologically, sociologically, anthropologically, and pathologically derived principles of nursing care. Developing in the students the capacity to understand biological principles is essential in

Figure 3: Broad conceptual framework – an example for nursing

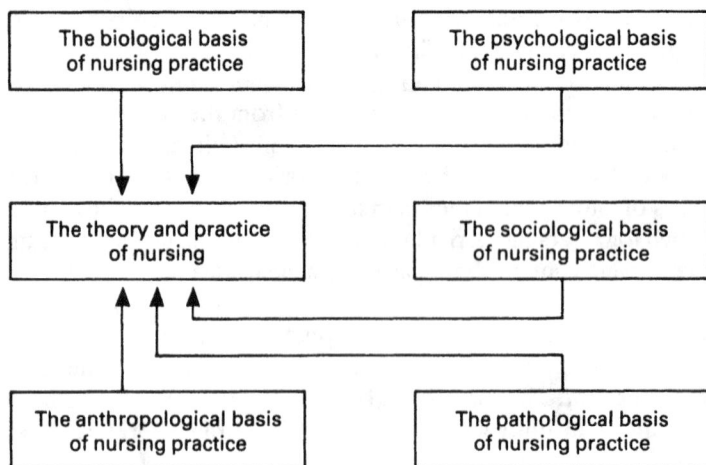

relation to deepening and broadening their understanding of the physical needs of the patient in health and disease. A theoretical and practical knowledge of human behaviour is required with a focus on the individual person, the individual in society, social systems and cultures, cultural differences and comparisons. With these perspectives the focus is on the person as a whole, his interaction with other individuals and the ways in which social, cultural and institutional arrangements have influence on health and disease. As the nursing profession becomes more concerned with holistic and individual approaches to care, and as the trend to the de-institutionalisation of care develops towards community and environmental health focus, a broader base of underpinning knowledge is needed for the study of nursing.

Nursing as a distinctive knowledge area in its own right is developing slowly from its present state of conceptual frameworks and models to the beginnings of potential theories to support practice. This specific nursing knowledge has a sufficiently recognisable outline to form a broad frame of reference for the content of the curriculum. As its incremental development continues it is necessary to identify it as the central focus of the content and the organisational centre to which the integration is directed. The functional activities of nursing must be the central focus in the frame of reference and the theory and practice that constitute nursing as a unique form of health care must be included.

Organisational schemes of work for integration

We have seen that when attempting to integrate content it is important to know exactly what has to be integrated and what the expected outcomes are to be. The actual detailed arrangements can to a large extent be developed through what has become known as the integrating schemes of work. Aims, objectives, content, learning experiences, and evaluation procedures have to be assembled into an organised and meaningful state. This organisation has also to take account of scope, sequence, and continuity, using vertical and horizontal relationships which together create a total operational picture.

Ideally the areas of the content should relate to one another horizontally and vertically so that materials and activities can be expanded progressively into larger and more meaningful patterns. The horizontal relationships in the organisation of content takes into account the consideration of scope and integration. This horizontal relationship often cuts across more than one subject area and links to teaching and learning activities and some assessment and evaluation of student learning. The vertical relationship is more concerned with the sequence of events and the order of progression through the subject matter. Continuity, which is part of the vertical relationship, seeks to link smoothly each successive student experience in a subject area and to maintain a state of continuous progression through the course content. Continuity attempts to link by building each new experience successively from its preceding one. For the student this should mean a smooth journey through each element of a subject.

Bruner (1960) developed the idea of 'the spiral curriculum' where the students 'come round' through a series of themes and return to familiar concepts and ideas which are presented at increasingly higher levels of difficulty and which the curriculum presents using a variety of samples (Bruner, 1960, pp 52–4). In this approach students revisit familiar theory and practice but each successive experience builds up and each topic is gone into more broadly and at greater depth and difficulty. The emphasis is not just on reinforcement by replication but is on dealing with material at higher levels of understanding with each successive learning experience encountered by the students. In this manner each experience reinforces the previous one and also extends it.

A similar approach has been offered by Greaves (1984, pp 65–6), where the nursing process can be revisited at different year levels in the nursing curriculum. In the first year of training the emphasis is on a basic level application of the nursing process using standard care plans in individualised care contexts. In the second year a higher level of application of the process is introduced which focuses on greater complexities of technical, behavioural, and social skills, and using more sophisticated problem-solving approaches and evaluation procedures. In the third year of training theoretical frames of reference from various nursing models are used within the nursing process and a much broader dimension of study is developed to increase process applications to broad specialities.

The organisational principles of integration through the use of

Figure 4: An example of an integrating scheme of work

	Objectives	Nursing theme	Biological basis	Psychological basis	Socio-anthropological basis	Methods	Student activities
1.	Conceptual analysis and definitions	Definition of pain	Endogenous pain control mechanisms	Pain perception	Pain as a cultural value	Lecture ↓	Forward preparation using work book and study guide
2.	Identify type location and quality of pain	Assessment of individual patients pain	The neuro-physiological gate control theory of pain	Pain expression	Cross-cultural variation in pain	Tutorial ↓	Literature search and pre-reading assignment
3.	Identify degree of intensity, nature of onset, duration and precipitating factors	Identifying the nature of pain – origin and distribution	Pain threshold	Pain and personality	Environmental influences on pain control	Seminar (Sequence)	Practical exercise on patient assessment and communication approaches
4.	Identify any cultural or environmental factors	Factors which aggravate the pain	Pain tolerance	Attitudes to pain and pain control		Inter-disciplinary team teaching on one 1/2 day (theme pain)	Supervised practice in the care of selected patients
5.	Identify any significant behavioural changes	Factors which reduce the pain	Measurement of pain	Pain and suggestibility			
6.	Plan and provide any appropriate nursing interventions	Communicating with patients about pain	Establishing principles in the management of pain control	The pain–anxiety relationship			
7.	Teach the patient pain relief methods	Planning of nursing care to control and reduce pain		Behavioural methods of pain control			
8.	Consider research studies of pain relief	Implementation of care to control and reduce pain					
9.	Determine care evaluation procedures	Evaluating the effects of care					

Horizontal progression — Scope

Vertical sequence — Continuity

integrating schemes of work can be seen in Figure 4. Such schemes are often referred to as scope and sequence charts and they are useful in presenting the context.

Problem solving and integration

The focus of study are problems which require an input from a number of subjects and can be distinguished from a core approach in that no one subject usually has a central thread. The problems are often related to major issues of concern which for nursing might be such things as pain, communications, health education and compliance, the extended role of the nurse, implementing new care approaches, and the use of the nursing process as a problem-solving approach to care. One of the main objectives of this approach is to encourage enquiry and to provide a stimulating learning environment using methods and approaches from a number of disciplines to help throw light on a problem. By bringing several course perspectives to bear on a specific problem the student learns to apply the principles of disciplines such as psychology and sociology and make a contribution to the problems of nursing practice.

Projects and assignments

Problems may be set through projects or assignments providing that the necessary advanced organisation directs the students into an enquiry approach. In effect a distinctive teaching–learning method is being used in such a way that the students have to address several subject areas in an attempt to deal with problems intrinsic to the exercise. For nursing applications the nature of the assignments should encourage the development of such characteristics as data identification and collection, the ability to analyse, synthesise, and evaluate activities of nursing care and their effects on patients. The students should be guided into developing problem-solving approaches that will help them formulate a procedure for tackling problems based on traditional scientific method.

Resource units

Integration has been attempted through the general idea of resource-based learning. This system encourages progressive ideas and a flexible use of a wide range of resources. The term resources includes teachers (generally as facilitators and consultants), educational technology and a whole range of learning materials, a mix of independent and collaborative learning approaches including the use of computer technology, learning packages, work books, study guides, extensively linked library resources with an active learning climate, and easy access to teaching staff. The whole approach tends to have an 'open' learning climate and favours an adult approach to learning with some considerable emphasis on self-paced learning. For this approach to be used successfully as an integrating scheme it usually requires central themes or a main subject ideology into which eclectic areas can be applied. It must of course be accepted that resource units usually based in libraries or computer services departments or in combination with each other are generally part of the curriculum materials used on most courses.

The distinctive thing about resource-based learning as a curriculum integrator is that it should by definition integrate the course content through its methodology of learning. A final word on the question of integration for nursing courses. The developing body of nursing knowledge must be the central focus towards which integration is directed. The intentions and purposes of the nursing curriculum should be integrated to the content along with the learning and teaching methodology to be used in the course of study. Evaluation which is to be considered at length in the chapter on evaluation also needs to be looked at as a potential factor in assisting in integration. In order to secure an organised pattern in the curriculum the following check lists are offered as a means to focus on a planning format to ensure that the required characteristics of scope, sequence, and integration are identified. (See Tables 1, 2 and 3).

Table 1: Check list for scope

---

(1) Move from general to specifics, universals to particulars, concrete to abstract, the known to the unknown.
(2) What are the major areas of knowledge to be included?
(3) Is the subject matter chosen for the unit worthwhile?
(4) Is the subject matter relevant and appropriate?
(5) At what level of intellectual and practical difficulty will the material be offered?
(6) What are the needs of the learner? What do they need to learn in terms of skills, attitudes and knowledge?
(7) Is there a need to bring in expertise from outside?
(8) What will be the major practical applications in clinical areas?
(9) Which resources and technology are needed and available?
(10) Consider previously established traditional approaches that have stood the test of time and may or may not be of value to the new curriculum.
(11) Which texts, reading, and general curriculum materials are needed? Do present resources provide these?
(12) Which assessments, examinations, and other forms of evaluation are appropriate for inclusion?
(13) Identify potential external constraints, finance, statutory requirements, work placements, Government and Health Authorities.

Table 2: Check list for sequence

---

(1) Consider the inherent logic of the subject matter and maintain that logic with the sequence. Unfold the subjects naturally as a logical development.
(2) Consider the historical and chronological development of material if these factors are appropriate to the subjects.
(3) Consider the difficulty of the material? Which elements are hardest to learn and do the students have any prerequisite knowledge?
(4) At which appropriate points in the sequence of material will students be ready to learn?
(5) Are there any factors of immediacy? The value and usefulness of individual topics at particular points in the curriculum.
(6) Maintain an appropriate sequence of objectives to content and methods. What can in general be learned at different levels by the students?
(7) When should particular subjects and topics be offered? At what point should they be started and completed?
(8) How many recurring experiences are needed at increasing levels of difficulty?
(9) Is there a need to present material in differing forms of application as new perspectives?

(10) Is there a need to sequence in periods of emphasis to develop over-learning with particularly important or difficult topics?

(11) Is there a need to increase periods of 'duration' for topics when there is increased complexity demanded in the learning?

Table 3: Check list for integration

(1) Identify the major themes, sub-themes, and subject threads.

(2) Develop an appropriate horizontal structure of progression.

(3) Develop a vertical structure of progression.

(4) Maintain continuity with a natural unfolding of subject areas.

(5) Develop commonality by matching appropriate elements of different subject areas that have similarity and things in common.

(6) Develop assessment procedures that cut across subject areas as well as ensuring testing of individual subject areas.

(7) Make use of teaching methods and learning experiences to integrate subjects by using appropriately seminar, project, problem solving or learning packages, where several subject elements are brought together within a given theme.

(8) Use the nursing process and appropriate nursing models to integrate elements from different subject areas, such as biology, psychology, and sociology.

It is clear that the integration of the curriculum for nursing education can be dealt with in a variety of ways, including the use of core curricula, broad conceptual frameworks, nursing models, and the nursing process. Whatever the general approach is to be, its effectiveness will in the final analysis, be dependent on the extent to which the curriculum designers can identify the order, structure, scope and balance, which is necessary to produce an appropriate unified whole. In effect it is concerned with 'putting it all together' in the best possible way to ensure that the curriculum provides the student of nursing with a unified view of nursing and related health care knowledge, rather than a segmented one. It is important that the principles of curriculum organisation presented in this chapter are seen to reflect a concern for the learner as well as for the subject matter to be developed. Within the curriculum for nursing there should be many opportunities to relate subjects such as nursing, health, life, and behavioural sciences, so that an integrated view is obtained by the students. In applying the essential principles of curriculum organisation through the use of scope, sequence, continuity, and integration, there must be a concern for the learner as well as a concern for the subject matter to be developed. This will be achieved by using an organising framework that gives systematic direction to the education of the students and encourages coordination of the efforts of the teachers involved. The task of organising the curriculum towards meaningful unity is a difficult and formidable one. Not withstanding the complexities of subject matter, systematic organisation is a vital process which requires very careful attention throughout the development of the curriculum.

5

Methodology in the Nursing Curriculum

The word method in the curriculum is concerned with the ways in which the content is learned and the approaches used to bring that learning about. The methods include the nature and form of teaching and the means and ways to provide and create the necessary learning experiences for the students. It includes the identification of methods to be used, the selection, preparation and use of appropriate materials, and the organisation of planned learning experiences. Teaching focuses on the delivery of these and the planned interaction between teachers and learners that will result in desirable learning outcomes. The methods also include the total range of curriculum resources which, when effectively used, assist the teacher and the learner to facilitate the learning concerned.

TEACHING AND LEARNING ENVIRONMENT

Teaching is much more than simply instructing students or transferring formal knowledge and information to them, and learning is much more than simply listening to the teacher and attempting to absorb these things. Both teaching and learning are activities and the methodology of the curriculum should be concerned with the most appropriate ways of organising these activities so that the students are in a rich and stimulating learning environment. The learning climate should be free from petty authoritarian restrictions and the sort of suffocating constraints that have been placed on the educational diet of nurses in the past. It is essential that the learning environment for nurses is one that is appropriate for adult learning to take place in. This does not mean a situation where there is no discipline or control, but one where the discipline is within the students' approach to the learning itself and the subjects and knowledge disciplines being studied. The essential approach is one where the learner and teacher are able to collaborate closely in a learning climate of mutual respect.

Too often in the past the nursing curriculum has produced a highly competitive learning environment in which undue emphasis was placed on the mastery of isolated facts and fragmented information, which was tested by a 'rite of passage' typified in the apprenticeship system used. The feeling that the students were 'racing through' the curriculum in the formal blocks and modules in order to get back to their patients and the work ethic responsibilities of the wards has mitigated against the development of a student-centred learning environment. At the same time and for similar reasons the learning environment in the clinical settings had developed as a trial and error situation in which the students are socialised into the traditional and often ritualised nursing practices of previous generations of nurses. The 'hoops and hurdles' characteristics of nurse training clearly illustrated by Salvage (1985), reflects the use of a methodology within which the curriculum of the past has never remotely approached the idea of an educational experience for the students.

The narrow training focus had been characterised through a pragmatic expectation of the students being prepared for a heavy contribution to the work in the wards. The trained staff in many instances had expected the students to come to the wards already possessing the skills that the students thought they had come to learn. It is clear that in the past and to a large extent at present, the learning environment has been recognised by nurse teachers as the formal environment of the school classrooms, which is quite illogical in a traditional training curriculum when the skills of nursing patients are acquired in the clinical areas that the students are allocated to. The clinical settings and the formal learning environment of the classrooms are both complementary aspects of the total learning arena of the curriculum and each must receive the same emphasis as focal centres of learning for students of nursing. There must be equal amounts of forward planning and involvement by teachers in both ward and classroom teaching and the teachers of nursing should be concerned with the conditions of learning for both areas.

With the current demise of the clinical teachers who generally have been badly used as teacher–practitioners in the past there is a need to reskill nurse tutors in practical nursing expertise through formal preparation wherever new curriculum is being designed and implemented. For a practising profession such as nursing it is inconceivable that students of nursing are not taught by practitioners of nursing who have current and up-to-date experience. Nurse tutors are part of the resources of the curriculum and should be prime movers in the creation of the total learning environment for the students and in order to do this they need to be capable of operating as teachers in both the classroom and their own fields of practice.

What can the clinical environment offer the curriculum?

Let there be no doubt in any nurse teacher's mind that the skills of nursing can only be learned by students in the reality of real nursing contexts in real patient situations. Students can be taught nursing in classrooms and a great deal of the essential theory needs to be taught there, but the learning of nursing, the *raison d'être* as far as the curriculum is concerned, has to be learned in clinical settings.

What should be taught to the students and which learning experiences do the students need to learn? This question is an important one as far as the clinical learning environment is concerned. As students are allocated to learning experiences for set periods of time to gain specific experience it is important that they derive the most benefit from the experience available. Basic skills and knowledge need to be developed all the way through a student's training but when special experience of a particular type of care is only available in one clinical setting and the student may not meet it again, then that experience becomes one of the priorities. The experience offered to the students in a specific clinical placement has to have special meaning for them and clearly needs to be made more than simply a number of weeks' experience or just a contribution from the students to the work requirements of the ward. In effect what it has to be is an exciting and fulfilling learning experience within which the students can progressively improve their patient care skills and develop a growing ability to provide patient-centred care. The clinical environment is ideal for the presentation to the students of naturally occurring nursing care problems to be identified and dealt with in the real situation. The curriculum needs to present the students with all the functions, procedures, and range of nursing care available in the area so that they can be open to analysis regarding their use, purpose and effectiveness. Each ward or department is a potential learning area and has to identify what it can offer to the students as essential learning opportunities.

Within the clinical learning environment contact with the patient is the most desirable of the learning opportunities available to the student and needs to be seen as the major focus of the curriculum in the wards and departments. The patient and his environment with its resources make up the true learning place for the students. The patient presents for the students an accurate and recordable source of clinical data. He represents the physical, behavioural, and social phenomena as effects of his illness or condition which he shows through his actions and responses to his treatment and nursing care. He is less predictable in his reactions to his condition and care than the medical and nursing textbooks would have us believe, yet his reactions are true and accurate and are an indisputable source of information and knowledge for the student to learn from. The patient will talk about his views and he is a totally reacting individual and constitutes the most readily available set of potential measurements of the quality of nursing care. As a part of the learning environment of the curriculum the patient surely is the most valuable and singularly important contribution to the student's learning experience.

Perhaps the most significant influences on the students next to the patient are the ward sister and other trained nursing staff that the students have frequent contact with. For good or bad their influence has a considerable and major lasting effect on the development of students, and their future values, beliefs and attitudes, as well as the technical competence acquired under their supervision. Bandura (1971) has demonstrated the powerful learning influence that can be developed through the effects of 'role modelling' by close contact with the ideal model. The ward sister and the staff nurse are potentially the most valuable role models for the students and with good quality sisters and staff nurses who demonstrate high levels of skill and competence in direct patient care and patient care management, are the ideal role model for students to emulate. When these levels of skills are linked to a genuine desire to influence the students by planned guidance, careful supervision, and appropriate teaching, the students respond positively. They are stimulated by such role models and respond with enthusiasm and interest, and a desire to acquire the characteristics and competencies themselves. They become more conscientious and disciplined in learning and develop a motivation and trust under the influence of the role model on which to base their own personal development as nurses. The selection of wards and clinical departments within which there are good role models and appropriate learning experiences available for students and a commitment to providing a teaching input is an essential requirement for the clinical learning environment.

Reid (1985) has recently researched the clinical learning environment and developed appropriate and effective tools for assessing their potential effectiveness as learning areas. Curriculum planning teams should address themselves to the findings of this research when considering the selection of wards and departments for possible learning situations. It is also important that the trained nursing staff have the necessary teaching and assessment skills to enable them to make a contribution to their students learning. Part of the planning of curriculum is concerned with making sure that all the people making a teaching input to the courses have the necessary skills and teaching abilities and this may mean arranging for the necessary staff development in order to meet this requirement.

The technology and equipment of wards and departments are also essential learning resources for the students. As clinical areas become increasingly specialised it is necessary for students to become familiar and competent with the equipment and technology that they meet within a specific period of clinical experience. The ability of students to identify, select and use equipment in nursing interventions is best developed in clinical settings rather than classroom settings and this is true of all clinical data and observational materials and techniques. Letting the students see and handle materials whenever possible rather than simply talking about them during a discussion or preceding or following a demonstration is essential to support the teachers' descriptions and explanations. Telling students about things has to be supplemented by showing them and allowing them to use as many senses as possible. The ability of students readily to identify and manipulate equipment for nursing purposes involves the use of touch, dexterity, vision and the development of a total familiarity which only comes from guidance in handling, identifying parts, and being questioned on function and range of use. The technical and physical skills of nursing care are clearly part of the clinical learning environment for the curriculum, as are the behavioural and social skills of patient interaction and interpersonal communication. The ability of students to converse with and communicate effectively with patients can only realistically be acquired in the clinical setting with real patients and in real nursing contexts. Opportunity to do so has to be engineered into the learning environment of the wards and departments where students are placed for experience.

The current concern for developing individualised nursing care approaches through the use of the nursing process also can only be learned effectively in clinical areas where these approaches are being used. It is irresponsible and irrational to expect students to acquire the skills and application of nursing process knowledge in a ward climate where the normal way of operating is through the ritualised use of regimented task and procedure. All areas designated as learning experience areas for the students must be organising nursing care using individualised approaches and be selected for inclusion as part of the learning environment on the understanding of this requirement.

THE CLASSROOM ENVIRONMENT AND THE NURSING CURRICULUM

The traditional classroom and practical room format in schools of nursing characterises the formal nature of nurse training and its knowledge transmission ideology. It also reinforces the idea of socialising students into the traditional roles, attitudes and beliefs of the 'trained' nurse and sets out to replicate the cultural and traditional values of nursing. Whilst this is not necessarily a bad thing in itself there has been an over-concentration on training in the narrow sense of the word and an under-emphasis on the presentation of an educational climate for the preparation of nurses to take place in. Too often in the past the over-riding concern has been to prepare students for an immediate contribution to the nursing work force in the wards and departments imposing a historically-derived commitment on the nurse educators in which the hospitals have always had a vested manpower interest. In the schools a situation has been created in which the prior concern has been with equipping the student with the basic abilities necessary to enable them to fit into the working environment the students would soon find themselves in, not for learning or necessarily educational reasons, but to become part of the hospital organisation.

The traditional pedagogic teaching arrangements common to most nursing courses have tended in the past to fit fairly well to the narrow training approaches used and the compliant student body generally responded as passive participants. The approach necessary for the present day student body of nurses needs to be one based more on the 'andragogic' model developed by Knowles (1980) and successfully used in a wide range of adult educational settings. This model breaks away from the authoritarian classical didactic approach in which the main method of teacher–student contact is through exposition, class teaching, and the maintenance of a teacher-dominated environment. With an andragogical (adult) perspective the tendency is towards student-centred approaches and a participative learning climate in which learning becomes the central focus rather than teaching.

The general characteristics of the learning environment are a flexible use of a variety of methods and the creation of learning experiences that encourage student activity. The teacher–student relationship is transactive with teachers working more with the students in a collaborative way. Learning resources are valued, inquiry is encouraged and the creative element of the teacher role is developed through attempts to facilitate student learning. For the students the possibility of a self-fulfilling educational experience is much more likely and individual student learning responsibility is nurtured. With such a learning method emphasis, it is essential that the teachers concentrate early in the course on enabling students to 'learn how to learn' using a full range of learning resources for both individual and small group contexts. The andragogic approach should not be confused with the so called 'romantic-progressive' approach of the 1960s used in primary schools which valued a child centred focus, discovery methods and freedom based on a *laissez-faire* approach. The adult learning focus seeks to produce a planned set of learning activities for the student using appropriate learning methods and curriculum materials which encourage the development of responsibility for one's own learning and self-development, which will be carried on long after a particular course of study has been completed.

The emphasis so far in this chapter has been with the nature of the learning environment and its importance for the nursing curriculum and the suggestion that an adult learning approach be used. An over-view of general methods is now offered with the assumption that certain principles of methodology will help significantly in the organisation of the curriculum for the purpose of enabling learning to occur in the adult environment.

GENERAL PRINCIPLES FOR SELECTING LEARNING EXPERIENCES

Learning experiences should allow the students to achieve the expected learning outcomes and for any objective the student requires, opportunity to practise the kind of behaviour implied by the objective. For instance, problem-solving skills to be acquired by the student can only realistically be learned in a problem-solving situation and it is the responsibility of the teacher to provide appropriate problem-solving situations in nursing situations that present the circumstances necessary for the student to solve problems.

It is also important that the students are ready to learn from any particular learning situation that they are to be involved in. In other words the student must be in a state of readiness or in a state of predisposition to learn. This means that any forward preparation by the student for a particular learning session has previously been carried out. Such preparation allows the student to familiarise herself with the material to be learned and includes appropriate reading materials, review of learning objectives concerned, and any source materials that may be appropriate including such things as patient observations and patient care data. In effect the student is actively encouraged to come to a learning session sufficiently prepared to take an active part in the proceedings. The teacher role in this instance is to advise and guide the student in her forward planning and is an example of facilitation or enabling the student to be ready for her part in her own learning experience. The learning experience must also be a relevant one for the student and have as far as possible a chance of application in the clinical setting. This factor of immediacy is important for student nurses and a link to patient care should be developed as often as possible. The learning experience should be a satisfying one for the student in that she can experience some obvious learning gain and a positive outcome. The good teacher will always produce a learning experience for the student where a successful outcome is likely or the student is allowed to experience some advancement in ability.

The selection of a learning experience needs also to be concerned with developing the thinking or cognitive skills of the student. Getting nurses to think in nursing situations is important so that knowing why something is done is of equal concern as knowing how to do something for a patient. Thinking as part of learning behaviour usually involves relating more than one or two ideas; it includes thinking critically about the nursing care to be given and the nurse using her knowledge and skills to deal not just with an isolated activity of care but with the total care of the patient. This requires the use of both inductive and deductive thinking. With inductive thinking the student considers the available observed data of the patient and works towards a generalisation of the main problems. In the deductive approach the student uses known theoretical generalisations and applies a theory to bring light to observed data. Both forms of thinking are part of logical thought and in any complex nursing situation both forms can be used. In the organisation of nursing care using the nursing process where assessment, planning, implementation and evaluation are concerned, cognitive thinking is as important as the psychomotor and interpersonal skills of nursing. In order to develop these thinking skills the selected learning experiences should allow the student to use these forms of thinking and the nurse teacher needs to create learning situations within which the skills can be developed in direct relationship to the nursing care of patients.

Problem solving as a learning method involves the use of a cognitive approach by the students. The problem should be of the sort that requires the relating of a number of facts and ideas in order to develop the best solutions, and they should also be the type by which the solutions are not necessarily available in text books. The student needs to learn how to identify problems which relate directly to patient care and which might already exist for the patient, or may be potential problems for the patient.

Learning experiences are required which help the student to acquire knowledge using their own logical thought processes rather than simply receiving information from the teacher. For the student, information seeking is essential as is the development of abilities to interpret and use the information in patient care contexts. It is important for nurse teachers to see the value of setting up learning experiences in which specific information necessary to solve particular problems is available and can be acquired by the students at the same time as they are expected to solve the problems. The nursing process is an ideal problem-oriented learning tool and if this process is to be used effectively in the practise of nursing, continuous opportunities need to be given to students so they may acquire the appropriate skills involved. The nurse teachers have to nurture in their students problem-solving attitudes to nursing care and provide learning experiences with a problem-oriented basis. The need is to develop in the students a spirit of inquiry, a need to question, appraise and evaluate critically the circumstances of a patient's problems and at the same time use initiative in resolving those problems. The nurse teacher should guide and facilitate the learner to think in terms of solving a patient's problems through helping the student to organise and direct care to meet his individual and personal needs. This means helping the student to develop a conscious desire to obtain first hand information by encouraging and guiding searching activity. The nurse who can evaluate situations critically, and make decisions based on observation and inquiry, is more likely to be successful in handling the problematic nature of the nursing process when it is applied to nursing care. This does not mean that all previous traditional nursing practices are necessarily invalid or suspect. It does however mean that existing practices should be adapted to the individual needs of patients to de-ritualise their use and to develop in new students the idea of creativity in nursing and the use of a more scientific approach for proposing solutions to care problems. For a detailed approach to the nursing process and the application of problem solving see Greaves (1984, pp 66–73).

The following format is offered for guiding the creation of problem oriented learning activities:

(1) Give the student a solvable problem or enable the students to seek a problem related if possible to direct patient care.

(2) Help the student to state and to delimit the problems by reducing them to writing through a written statement of the nature of the problem. Question the student on her knowledge of the patient and whether she has identified a valid problem or not. Are both the nurse and the patient agreed that a problem exists? This is important because defining a problem involves both the patient and the nurse.

(3) Help the student to find any needed information which may relate to the patient's physical, psychological or social needs, or has implications for his responses to his condition or management of his care. The student should be encouraged to view the patient as a primary source of information and evidence, and secure knowledge by observing, communicating, and using any recorded information from observational and care data. The student then organises and collates the information into a logical order.

(4) Help the student to interpret and analyse the information data by attempting a critical evaluation. The student should assess the patient's needs in the light of the information and evidence she has collected. Essential and non-essential data should be identified and irrelevant material discarded. The nurse teacher discusses the data with the student and questions her to develop understanding and meaning.

(5) Opportunity should be provided for the student to implement and test her ideas and define a course of action to deal with the patient's problem, and from assessment of the available evidence devise and set nursing objectives on which the subsequent care can be based. A nursing care plan can be produced or the existing plan modified so that additional objectives can be achieved.

(6) The nurse teacher and student discuss the care plan and the student implements the additions to care. Both teacher and student carefully review the additional care through further observation and seek to anticipate any further needs. The patient's responses to further care are carefully evaluated.

Securing information necessary to understand particular patient problems by using principles of observation, cognitive thinking, and available evidence are clearly more important than nurse teachers simply giving information to students. For the student, information retrieval and analysis is highly preferable to information receiving, and for the teacher information seeking by the student is of more value than situations where the information is given by the teacher. Acquiring the ability to use information is also more important than students merely attempting to memorise data. This important inquiry characteristic of problem solving and the development of the ability to organise data into meaningful relationships develops necessary discriminative skills in the student and the ability to organise effective personalised care for the patient. Such approaches are valuable as appropriate learning experiences for students of nursing and need to be increasingly incorporated into the curriculum both in clinical learning, and classroom environments.

TEACHING AND LEARNING TECHNIQUES
IN THE CURRICULUM

Teaching and learning techniques need to have a clear relationship to the subject matter of the curriculum and the correct choice of approaches is highly significant for the design of nursing courses. In making choices concerning curriculum methods two essential factors seem to be *a priori* in the overall scheme of things. Firstly that the teaching and learning are student centred, and secondly that the content dealt with is patient care centred or has potential application to patient care in some way. Student centredness as a desirable theme in the nursing curriculum has been reviewed previously in this chapter along with the idea of an 'andragogical' or adult learning approach. Incorporating such approaches should still allow for a variety of teaching and learning methodology which can provide an adequate basis for both direct and vicarious learning experiences. The essential feature is that the students are allowed to learn by experience and, the process of learning itself is the essential concern rather than over-reliance on direct formal teaching. In general direct experience is preferable to vicarious experience but this depends on the level of difficulty and the newness of the subject material being learned.

Nursing as a practising profession clearly lends itself to direct experience and patient centred approaches are ideal ways of meeting this relationship. Nursing students as relatively mature adult learners are mentally mature enough to apply generalisations and to handle theoretical abstractions by vicarious experience, if they have had enough direct experience related to clinical areas within which they are working. Whether experiences are direct or vicarious a patient care orientation is critical and can help to provide for both intellectual and practical skills development.

Patient centred teaching and learning involves the use of methods and materials which are directly concerned with understanding the patient, his needs and the care he will require. The patient is always the focus or central consideration in the learning experience to be provided. The approach may draw on other subject areas which are supportive in understanding nursing but the use of supporting subjects is on an eclectic basis in which only the relevant elements are studied and not necessarily the whole discipline. Application to nursing care of the supporting subject material is the reason for its inclusion in the learning experience, whether it be a direct experience or a second order or vicarious experience. In the patient-centred approach there is a triangulation of inter-relationships between teacher, student, and the patient (see Figure 5). This can be seen in direct experience in the clinical setting where the teacher functions as nurse and teacher or teacher practitioner and demonstrates, describes, and explains the care of the patient. The patient is the focus of instruction and the patient's environmental context becomes the learning environment for the student. The student is actively involved in the care of the patient, and the communications and interpersonal relationships are three way. The patient-centred teaching and learning approach makes use of patient-centred nursing care a different but similar concept which relates to the individualised care of the patient, and is diametrically opposed to the ritualistic task-orientated care which is inspired by procedure.

If patient-centred teaching and learning are to work correctly, procedures, skills and tasks have to be seen in terms of their effects on the individual patient through the application of

Figure 5: The triangulation of patient–centred teaching and learning

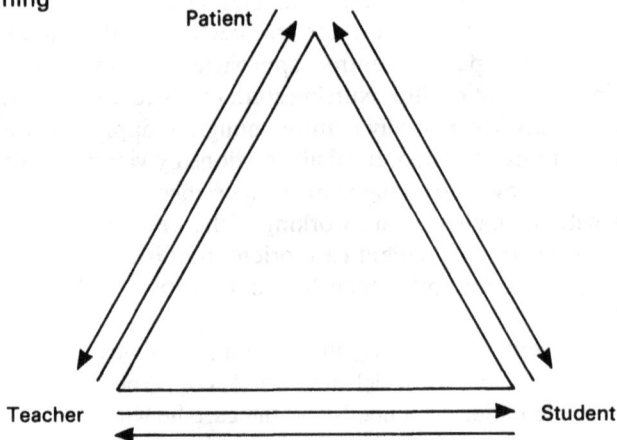

personalised care. The type of teaching methods appropriate to help learners grasp the essentials of patient-centred care are direct bedside teaching and learning as part of on-going nursing care, clinical nursing conferences, and clinical nursing rounds.

PATIENT-CENTRED TEACHING AND LEARNING: DIRECT EXPERIENCES

Clinical nursing conference

The idea here is to confer and discuss to provide an exchange of information and expert opinion about the nursing care of a patient. The conference may include learners and practising nurses, the ward sister, and the nurse teacher. The method involves reviewing the care given to the patient and his response to that care. The learning objectives are:

(1) to provide opportunity to evaluate the nursing care of the patient and to discuss possible solutions to problems and plan further changes for care,

(2) to increase the quality of nursing care,

70

(3) to increase the level and quality of communication between nursing staff in the care of the patient,

(4) to provide a learning experience for students and to create a closer teaching and learning inter-relationship in patient care contexts.

The conference involves oral reporting, discussion and exchange of information and views about the on-going care of a patient, and the student participation is actively encouraged. The patient can be present in suitable instances for part of the time and if circumstances are not suitable for patient participation, nursing notes and observational data can be used for analysis and evaluation. The learning experience is essentially discussional with a focus on the total care of the patient, specific nursing care, observations and recorded data and their implications, the patient reactions, response to care, and progress. The medical and surgical treatment and consequences regarding how they relate to and effect the nature of nursing care to be given. Evaluation and modification of nursing care are the key factors in the learning exercise and include the solving of patient-care problems. Learner preparation for these sessions is important and they should be directed into forward organisation through pre-reading and general preparation for active participation.

Clinical nursing rounds

Another useful direct experience approach is through the use of the teaching–learning round. This allows the students direct patient contact and contact with the nurse teacher in a patient-centred environment. It is useful for teaching students patient communication and the development of good interpersonal relationships. In addition, nursing diagnosis, care planning and evaluation can be considered and patient responses to care and the seeking of information from the patient. One or two students can be taken by the nurse teacher practitioner to visit a small number of carefully selected patients. To some extent the exercise is a problem-solving one or can be developed as such. The condition and response of the patient to his illness and nursing care can be the main theme and by effective informal questioning and the development of a dialogue with the student, they can be tested on their knowledge and application of that knowledge to the nursing care, treatments, the patient's disease process, associated physical problems, and general observational alertness. Patient dignity, ethical discretion, and guarded medical knowledge can be maintained in the hands of a sensitive and experienced teacher. The advantages of this type of teacher–learner–patient interaction is that the student's grasp of patient problems and nursing care can be evaluated during the session. Knowledge can be tested and gaps filled with immediate feedback and knowledge of results. The student is encouraged to improve her communication skills by observing the trained nurse teacher practitioner in action and seeing her operate as the role model in communication and demonstrating good quality interpersonal skills. The clinical and learning experience gained by the student from the teaching round can be further expanded later, away from the bedside in informal discussion.

Nursing procedures as direct learning experiences

Procedure is only a method used to provide a particular aspect of nursing care and the principles inherent in each procedure are much more important than any obsession with its detail at the expense of neglecting any specific circumstance which relates to the patient's individual and personal needs at the time. From a teaching point of view attention to making the student aware of the reasons why a particular procedure is used and understanding the total consequences for the patient in question is essential. Nursing procedures can and should be made meaningful to the student at the time they are taught within a patient-centred context with the technicalities kept flexible to meet the patient's needs. The teaching and learning of procedures needs to be deritualised and individual creativity encouraged. This can be done by maintaining principles and patient safety, but at the same time developing logic, sequence, and adaptability for individual patients. Specific procedures require learning within total nursing care contexts and can be taught and practised within a nursing process approach to care.

In addition to teaching the skills of the procedure itself as a technical activity, opportunity for incorporating and developing interpersonal and social skills should also be made for the student. The procedure in question may be only one of a number of nursing tasks required for the patient's total comfort and the teacher has to make the learner see the numerous aspects in any one caring situation and learning experience. In addition to teaching the skills of the procedure itself the learning experience requires to provide for the student the whole range of nursing requirements that the patient needs. This includes communication awareness and the ability for the student to express herself clearly in language the patient can understand. During a planned learning experience for procedure learning the situation is also an ideal one for extending the student's observational alertness and her ability to act on the implications of observations made. It is also the most effective time to help the student develop a correct and caring attitude within the development of her procedural skills, by cultivating the necessary personal qualities of gentleness, firmness, and correct manner which has a profound effect on the patient's willingness to comply. The nursing characteristics outlined here are only learned in the direct experience setting. They can be taught in the indirect experience environment of practical suites in the school of nursing and such vicarious experience is useful but does not provide the reality of the direct experience. Obviously in selecting teaching and learning experiences in the curriculum to deal with specific content, the nature of the content has important implications for the type of methods to be used.

On-going teaching and learning of clinical nursing

The most singularly important curriculum strategy for learning nursing care is the nurse teacher's use of the clinical setting and the patients in it for teaching purposes. This involves the previously discussed patient-centred approaches to care and active student participation. It also involves planning for the effective use of the clinical environment and the identification of appropriate learning experiences. Creating successful learning experiences depends very much on planning rather than non-planning and the recognition and use of the resources of the clinical area to the best effect. Planning is directed at producing opportunities rather than relying on chance situations within which learning can take place.

Successful learning opportunities depend on the following criteria:

(1) working with specific objectives which are known to teacher and learner,
(2) working with the student and giving nursing care to patients,
(3) using the full potentialities of the clinical area including the direct care of patients,
(4) using ordered and logical approaches including individualised care and the principles of the nursing process,
(5) demonstrating nursing care by showing and doing with the student in attendance and assisting,
(6) describing, explaining, and interpreting, nursing care as it is carried out,
(7) closely guiding and supervising the student in the giving of nursing care,
(8) using theoretical applications of nursing care concepts,
(9) using theoretical applications of subjects which support nursing theory,
(10) developing the right attitudes and values in the students.

Given that teaching and learning in the clinical areas of direct experience should be planned rather than unplanned, one must assume that the activities involved are a set of pre-determined and organised learning experiences. In other words the learning is planned and guided by the nurse teacher practitioner and part of this concerns the setting up of the order and scope of what has to be taught in order that the desired learning takes place. This ordered design of clinical nursing learning activities should be planned and calculated to:

(1) identify student learning needs,
(2) formulate student learning objectives,
(3) identify what has to be taught and learned in terms of skills, knowledge, attitudes, and beliefs,
(4) select the correct learning experiences,
(5) identify, select, and use the most appropriate teaching methods,
(6) evaluate the student's gains in learning.

In effect have an ordered system of identifiable learning activities for the students and identify for them what they need to learn using a sequenced and logical approach. Within the experience area that the student has been allocated to she should be able to assess patients for care, set up care objectives, plan care delivery, implement the nursing activities, and evaluate their effects, by using systematic problem solving approaches to meet patient needs.The student should be able eventually to demonstrate her competence in a range of nursing care contexts by using the nursing process and identifying actual and potential patient problems by critically analysing the clinical, behavioural and social needs of the patient. She should acquire the range of abilities to plan the total scope of patient care, provide continuity in patient care, and integrate the individual nursing event into an ordered pattern of total nursing care. In addition she should be skilled in evaluating and continuously monitoring the effects of that care. All of these activities must be carried out as demonstrable performances which the teacher can assess for levels of competence.

Each student would require an outline study guide for the clinical area she is allocated to for specific learning experience. This can take the form of a clinical profile which can include the philosophy of the clinical unit, the type of patients nursed there, the forms of care dealt with and an outline of resources available. This would also include prescribed learning objectives, identified nursing skills to be mastered, knowledge, attitudes, and values to be acquired. Major themes of the profile could also include individualised care beliefs, individualised care approaches, fundamental and specialised nursing skills, and the use of nursing technology. Useful supporting theoretical outlines as principles and appropriate reading can be drawn from nursing, biological, behavioural, and social sciences. The fundamentals for planning a clinical nursing experience are highlighted by asking the following questions:

(1) What are the major purposes and intentions of the teacher?
(2) What will be the main learning objectives for the student?
(3) What skills, knowledge, attitudes and beliefs does the student need to acquire?
(4) What will be the end product of the clinical experience?

(5) Which teaching and learning methods are appropriate to bring about the desired learning in the student?
(6) Which sequence of learning is most useful?
(7) To what extent has the student achieved the necessary learning by the end of the learning experience?
(8) Design a basic teaching learning programme that will provide all the necessary learning experiences.

LEARNING NURSING AND NURSING RELATED EXPERIENCES IN THE CLASSROOM

It is not proposed here to give a detailed account of the many different teaching approaches. This has been admirably done by Quinn (1980), and Jarvis and Gibson (1986). It is proposed however to outline some of the more important requirements for the selection and use of teaching and learning methodology appropriate for the more formal classroom settings. The task then is to elaborate some of the criteria that can be of help in selecting teaching and learning experiences. Generally speaking there is no substantial evidence that any one teaching–learning approach has any significant advantage over others in that it is superior in bringing about learning. Principles of learning are useful as general guiding influences on the overall presentation of learning experiences, but learning theorists have made few attempts to transfer their findings into methods suitable for practising teachers. The majority of teachers tend to be highly influenced by teaching approaches they themselves were exposed to as students. Despite controversy in learning theory and in the application of that theory to real teaching situations there are some generally agreed principles which the curriculum should take account of with respect to the validity of methods and their suitability to fulfill learning requirements.

The following criteria are offered as guide-lines in selecting methods:

(1) Learning is an active process, therefore students of nursing should be actively involved as far as possible.
(2) Learning is more meaningful and proceeds more effectively if the student understands what she is learning. Therefore teachers must teach for meaning and learning

experiences should seek to develop meaning.

(3) The teaching approach and the learning activity must be appropriate to meet any given objective to be attained.

(4) The learning experience must be satisfying and relevant to the student's needs both in the immediate and long term, and the ability to learn is considerably affected by the student's individual goals, values and motivation.

(5) The learning experiences should be appropriate to her present attainments and predisposition to learn; the student must be ready for the learning in question.

(6) Many individual or different experiences can be used to obtain the same learning outcome and conversely the same learning experience may bring about several possible outcomes.

(7) Frequent repetition of response is important in learning skills.

(8) The greater the scope of experiences presented to the student, the more likely are generalisations and discrimination to occur.

(9) Similar teaching–learning experiences may produce different responses from different students because individual differences affect learning.

(10) The learning climate or group atmosphere has major implications which affect learning either positively or negatively depending on how the climate is influenced by teachers and students.

The selection of specific teaching methods is dependent on the job each method is intended to do. Lecture and formal talk approaches which are invariably teacher-dominated depend for their success on the individual skill and flair of the teachers involved. Such methods are necessary for the presentation of the main conceptual frameworks of content and the explanation of principles, relationships and overall frames of reference. The teacher is concerned with initiating interest and motivation for the subject and when this is done well students can become highly committed to the subject; conversely, however, in the hands of a poor lecturer the subject can be permanently destroyed for the student. Good all-round teachers do not always equal good lecturers. This particular method perhaps more than many others requires not only expertise in the subject matter but special expertise, style and flair, and considerable experience in handling the method successfully. Where these qualities in this method are available in staff then the lecture approach is a desirable one. It should of course be supplemented by tutorial or tutor-led discussion groups to develop the main themes of the lecture within which subject matter can be more carefully explained and analysed and students are able to participate much more actively in dialogue with the teacher. In the ideal situation particularly when a series of lectures and group tutorials are included in a course, they should be followed with group seminars which demand of the students fairly extensive preparation on the same subject themes dealt with in the formal lectures. In effect a link of methods and a variety of experiences are used to deal with a specific subject theme. The format is:

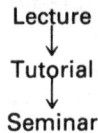

Lecture
↓
Tutorial
↓
Seminar

in a linear sequence with the amount of student participation progressively increasing from lecture to tutorial to seminar.

In the hands of good teachers these are well-tried methods and provide a sound learning experience for the students, but the depth of learning increases and the preparation required of the students is a learning experience in itself. Preparation for the tutorial and seminar components are ideal situations for students to secure information in support of topics under consideration and to identify relevant principles, theories, observations and evidence, which may support generalisations that are to be dealt with. The advantage of such forward preparation for the students is that they are encouraged to seek information rather than passively receive it, acquire ability to use information rather than simply to memorise it, organise information into meaningful relationships, and develop familiarity in using retrieval skills. Teachers guiding the students in these advanced organisers see the value of setting up the learning experiences in which information can be acquired at the same time as the students are learning to ensure their own participation.

Participation of the student in a range of recognised 'discussional type' group activities, whether these be teacher led or student led (with teacher in attendance), allows the student a number of advantages which help to develop their all-round learning ability. In the corporate activity of a discussion group where the students are seeking to put together knowledge, ideas, and opinions in a harmonious and collaborative manner, the members learn to learn from each other. They initially have to learn how to use the learning method itself (which is true of all learning methods), and the teacher acts as the major facilitation for this activity of learning to use the learning method. All discussional method approaches require careful planning both by the learner and the teacher. Discussion is not haphazard or aimless. It should be a carefully planned activity with clear objectives, and predictable rather than prescribed outcomes. The students learn to retrieve, analyse, assimilate, and apply information and the individual experiences of each student are pooled and their ability to express information verbally in a logical and constructive dialogue is developed. As well as clarifying their own reflective thinking and developing their general cognitive skills they learn to co-operate with others, seek facts, interpret information, recognise principles which apply to different situations, and readjust attitudes and beliefs in the light of new ideas perceived by themselves and others. The ability to lead and participate through discussion also helps the student nurse prepare for her interpersonal relationships with patients, doctors, family, and other members of her profession and the community.

Criteria for choice of teaching-learning methods in the curriculum

Talk. Informal, small to medium groups, short time span, introductions to longer sessions such as pre-practical/pre-clinical, demonstration, role-play, simulation, problem-solving, project preparation, study assignments, evaluation sessions, and the like.

Lecture and lecture variations. Formal talk approaches, scope of subject, frames of reference, development of main themes, summary and review of themes, illustration and clarification from expertise, development of significant information, motivation of students, demonstration of general issues and problems, disseminating new information and knowledge from personal research.

Discussional approaches. Type of learning methods involving discussion: Small group, teacher led and student led, group tutorial, seminar. Larger group, symposium, panel-type seminars, workshop groups, nursing care study groups, clinical group conferences.

Small group. Full student participation, face-to-face contact, development of social learning skills, personal and social adjustment, acquisition of forward planning skills, information retrieval, increased intellectual abilities and skills, increased cooperation, exchange of ideas, experience, opinions, values and beliefs. Encourages analysis, testing, and application of information, defining, interpreting, clarifying and summarising progress in problem solving. Experience and knowledge of the group used in defining and solving problems. Collaborative and independent learning (through preparation) encouraged and valued.

Large group. Active preparation and participation, often organised around problems (i.e. workshops), and presentation of organised subject matter. Discussion panel and audience, dialogue with experts on selected subjects within general themes. Symposium set programme of speakers in sequence on selected topics with audience participation and involving the use of a chairperson. Multi-disciplinary approach may be used. Up-to-date information and knowledge presentation and chance for audience to address expert opinion. Can be followed by small group discussion and feed-back to main group for comparisons and general analysis and review.

Demonstration. Teaching technique involving showing, explaining, and analysis followed by student practice, supervision, and evaluation. Highest probability of success in the clinical setting, can be used in the practical classroom or practice suite where success is limited through lack of credibility. Ideal for laboratory sessions in life and behavioural sciences. Skills analysis essential and time for reflective and analytic thought and student performance. Essential that the demonstrator is expert in the technique and that the procedure is transferrable to clinical setting applications. Direct application to real patients and real clinical settings important with immediate application and practice as soon as possible. Can by used to correlate theory and practice and complements role-modelling by the nurse teacher in the clinical setting. Demonstration *per se* can be part of a learning session within which other teaching methods are used, such as following a talk or preceding discussion or as a central element of a lesson.

Role-play and simulation. Spontaneous acting out of situations and problems as unrehearsed dramatic characterisation, has its origins in socio-drama and extensively modified for use in micro-teaching sessions. Valuable for developing empathetic insight and ability in interpersonal relationships and communication techniques. Simulation of a wide variety of potentially problematic nursing care situations. Requires general objectives and careful organisation for success involving clear general instructions to participants without rehearsal. Flexible arrangements needed with emphasis on short time-span, clear outcomes and spontaneous teacher and student analysis by general discussion.

Individualised and independent learning. The ultimate success of students in any educational system rests with their ability to learn as individuals and includes the acquisition of independent learning skills and the discipline of self learning and self development. The further one progresses in the system, the greater the emphasis and reliance on individual learning. As the nursing curriculum evolves to an increasingly higher level of intellectual and practical difficulty so the amount of individualised learning will expand proportionally as part of the established methodology.

This does not mean 'Good bye to the teacher' as far as the students are concerned. It does mean, however, a change in emphasis in the role of the teacher. The nurse teacher in the future will increasingly be involved in facilitatory activities of guiding, assisting, and the mentoral role in shaping students in the discipline and methods of self learning. This will not mean the abandonment of traditional approaches but an increasing supplementation of these with self learning as technology advances in these areas. Independent projects, learning packages, computer-assisted learning, will inevitably be an incremental development in curriculum methodology as education comes to terms with an increasingly computer-literate society.

There are several basic assumptions underlying the implementation of individualised approaches to learning within the nursing curriculum:

(1) For individualised approaches to be economically and operationally feasible, much of the material must be self instructional.

(2) The student nurse should be actively involved in the learning process.

(3) Not all students will require the same amount or kind of practice to acquire mastery of the same material.

(4) Different styles of learning require different techniques of instruction.

(5) Students will work at their own pace and power of learning.

(6) Students should be able with the help of the teacher to evaluate their own progress.

(7) Different learning materials will need to be made available to accommodate different learning styles.

(8) Students will need to become increasingly self-directing and self-initiating in their learning.

Nurse teachers will still maintain considerable face-to-face contact with students, particularly in the one-to-one personal tutorial situation and other small group and whole class contact. In effect the independent learning methods would be used complementary to the collaborative group work and whole class presentations. In general the implications are that self-instructional materials must be available for those students able to benefit from using them. Individualised learning approaches are dependent to a large extent on a full provision of self-learning resources as a resource unit within the school of nursing, and also on the provision of staff development for individual nurse teachers to acquire the necessary expertise. When a planning team opts for individualised learning as part of the curriculum methodology in a nursing course, implementing such change is dependent on the preparation of teaching staff to carry it out.

CURRICULUM MATERIALS

Curriculum materials are tangible resources used by the student and teacher, and when used correctly can assist in bringing about the desired learning in the student. These materials are not teaching techniques or methods, but are resources which directly support student learning and the conditions under which the learning takes place. The materials require design, testing, development, correct selection and usage, and evaluation of their effects in the curriculum. Examples of curriculum materials are: manuals, workbooks, study guides, learning packages, reference books, text books, advanced organisers, journal articles, learning programmes, computer learning programmes, library resources and information retrieval systems, films, audio-tapes, video-tapes, film-loops, models, specimens, vignettes, simulation games, clinical analysis records, and so forth.

The above list is not exhaustive or exclusive but gives an idea of the nature of the materials commonly in use, and the scope continues to increase. Developing materials for a curriculum involves some essential basic planning. Which materials are required and who will prepare them? Which students are they designed for and which teachers will make use of them? Are they commercially available or will they be made by the teacher. This is the sort of self questioning that needs to precede planning. The following are essential considerations:

(1) The type of learning the student is expected to develop.
(2) The context or environment in which the learning is to take place.
(3) Time available for the learning to be accomplished.
(4) The objectives to be achieved.
(5) The degree of difficulty of the material to be learned.
(6) Nature of skills to be developed, cognitive, affective, psycho-motor, or combinations of all.
(7) Readiness of the student for the materials to be used.
(8) Previous learning which preceded the present situation.
(9) Constraints likely to affect the quality of performance expected.

The development of curriculum materials is part of the normal curriculum development and as such is an on-going activity which is continuously open to monitoring and evaluation of effectiveness. The development of materials can be determined through the following process:

    (a) Prepare a preliminary development plan.
    (b) Identify the curriculum content (subject matter) to be dealt with.
    (c) Determine the learning objectives.
    (d) Identify any special curriculum materials needed.
    (e) Review the educational technology literature to identify which materials are available.
    (f) Identify materials lacking in the subject area to be dealt with.
    (g) Establish priorities for needed materials.
    (h) Decide which materials will need to be designed by the teacher.
    (i) Set up sub-committees of the planning team to consider materials design, testing, and implementation into course methodology.

One of the most useful and frequently-used area of materials is course work books and study guides. These often include the course philosophy, intentions and purposes, reading assignments, and self-learning activities or exercises that the student can participate in. The sequence of subject matter is of course followed and may be included by way of synopsis and or specific objectives included. Table 4 is offered as part of a worked example to indicate the possible format for a work book. The work book seeks to help students to make their way more easily through the different components of the course of study. It is designed to assist them to select and plan their own independent learning strategies and to increase at the same time their depth of understanding of the subject matter and its application. It is not offered as a substitute for the taught element of the course, but as an essential complement to it.

The work books may be divided into year, terms, modules, or subject unit, components usually relating to the sequences within which formally taught material is presented for class and group sessions. Units of material are usually divided into appropriate topics in progressive sequence, and topics relate to essential reading, learning activities, and further reading.

Table 4: Outline example of the essential areas of a workbook

---

Unit title: emerging theoretical frameworks for nursing practice

Learning objectives

(1) Compare, contrast, and analyse the various functional definitions of nursing,
(2) Define nursing as a concept, and differentiate by comparative analysis, interactionist-model, developmental-model, and systems-model,
(3) Use principles from the current conceptual frameworks of nursing to make theoretically-informed applications to nursing care,
(4) Identify the relevant elements of the disciplines basic to nursing and justify an eclectic use of this knowledge to support nursing practices,
(5) Describe the nursing process and analyse the discrete stages of the process for patient care applications,
(6) Use the nursing process in clinical nursing contexts.

Essential reading

Riehl and Roy (1980)
McFarlane (1980)
Colledge and Jones (1979)
Grovenor (1978)

Learning activities

(1) Define and write short notes on (a) processes, (b) taxonomies, (c) theory and (d) models.
(2) What is meant by the eclectic use of knowledge in nursing? State three examples and justify their use as basic to nursing.
(3) Make your own conceptual definition of nursing using no more than 50 words.
(4) Compare your definition with those of Henderson, Roy, and King.
(5) Compare and contrast: (a) problem solving theory, (b) systems theory, (c) nursing process, and (d) list characteristics of all three that can be applied to the nursing care of patients.

Further reading

Orem (1979)
Dickinson (1982)

Essential reading is that which the student must cover and is considered vital if the students are to derive maximum benefit from the course. It is important from a design point of view that there is an extensive cover of the topics and that students are aware that they need to be selective in their reading as some readings may cover the same themes. Further reading is that which the course team consider to be either supplemental to the essential reading, or which is specialist, or allows some students to pursue certain topics or themes in greater depth. Again the reading is selective and a wide range is presented from which students can make their own choices. Some of the references may link to a number of topics or themes and a good standard referencing system is essential making full retrieval details available in the workbook. The learning activities section is designed to help the students work through material and review their understanding of the various topics and reading assignments covered. These activities ideally should relate to both principles, and theoretical applications to practice wherever these are considered appropriate. To this end a considerable amount of student activity will be directed into sources of information and methods of retrieval. Activities can be organised to allow the students to approach topics in a problem solving way. It is of course essential for the students to receive facilitatory guidance from the nurse teacher in the use of the workbook even though the book may contain explicit notes on its use. In effect the students should be receiving guidance from the individual teachers who should be willing to work with their students as well as teach them.

Study guides are usually different from workbooks in that they focus as a guide to the course to be undertaken by the student. They do often include the philosophy of the course with an outline of intentions and purposes, and fairly precise learning objectives are offered. The major differences are that a synopsis of the full syllabus is given along with a possible outline model of the course. Full assessment and examination data is usually given and a review of the main practical applications and methods of testing student performance. Sample reading lists may also be included and an indication of the learning and teaching methods within which the course of study focuses.

6

Evaluation of the Curriculum in Nursing Education

Curriculum evaluation is one of the most important concepts in curriculum theory and practice and it is mainly concerned with finding out how effective the curriculum is and giving judgement on its quality. It is a process of delineating, obtaining and providing useful information for deciding among alternative actions (Stufflebeam, Foley, Gephart, Guba, Hammond, Merriman and Provus, 1971). It is essentially an active process, the major characteristics of which are the determination of value, worth, or merit. The evaluation process is normally viewed as a continuous activity rather than being discrete with beginning and end. Its main purpose is to bring about the continuous improvement of the curriculum and to facilitate its development. This is done through the selection and use of appropriate evaluation procedures. Evaluation procedures involve the systematic collection of comprehensive information about the effectiveness of the curriculum, the results of which can be acted upon to allow modifications to improve it.

A number of people may be and often are involved in evaluation and they make value judgements based on the findings of the procedures used. These judgements clearly have significant implications for decision-making about the curriculum and relate to many things. The most important of these are objectives, the realisation of the general philosophy and beliefs of the curriculum, how effectively the content has been dealt with, the extent and quality of the learning, the educational and vocational effectiveness, and the quality of management and use of resources. The broad scope of evaluation in nursing courses includes judgements being made of teacher and student performance, resources, materials and support services used within the school of nursing and its clinical learning areas which are used to implement and maintain the development of the curriculum. The ultimate product of the curriculum and the performance of the nurse produced will be a major focus as will be the means by which the end product was achieved. These are a few of the curricular elements that will be judged through the process of evaluation. The people who make these value judgements (the evaluators) include not only educators but also students, managers, administrators, curriculum specialists, employers, statutory and professional bodies, and the health consumers themselves.

TYPES OF EVALUATION PROCEDURE

Evaluation procedures applied to curriculum evaluation have been categorised as formative or summative and this broad distinction is accredited to Scriven (1967). Formative evaluation is the process which validates the curriculum during its on-going initial development phase. The results of such evaluation are acted upon fairly quickly and allow modifications to be made to the curriculum as it is implemented and during its initial implementation and continuous evolution. It is concerned with identifying and correcting weaknesses and generally with attempts to improve the curriculum. Most formative approaches operate in 'trial', 'monitor' and 'revise' cycles. The sequence involves trying out the curriculum materials, teaching approaches and learning experiences, systematically securing information about their effectiveness, and making the necessary adaptations to ensure the smooth running of the course.

Summative evaluation is normally carried out as an 'end-on' activity and its function is in its purpose of assessing a fully implemented course or curriculum programme. Evaluations carried out by statutory and professional bodies fall within the summative type, but similar approaches can be carried out internally by the institution itself or in fact by the course team. A major concern is with the 'capability' of the course to produce nurses who possess the appropriate standards of excellence both academically and as clinical practitioners. There is also concern for the efficient and effective use of educational resources and the general management of the curriculum. Results of summative evaluation are often concerned with whether a course will be adopted or continued and as such provide the basis for policy decisions about the future of a curriculum. The main differences between formative and summative evaluations lie within their purposes and their time of application. Formative evaluation is on-going and continuous and seeks to refine, adjust, and improve the course through an effective feed-back process. Summative evaluation is more concerned with a final judgement concerning the extent to which the intentions and purposes of the course have been met, and the degree to which it meets educational and professional needs. Has the curriculum in fact achieved these things that it set out to achieve?

Although the two main types of evaluation described clearly indicate distinctive purpose, both are used in the long-term development and improvement of the curriculum. At an internal level of evaluation, that is when the institution itself and its course teams are seeking to conduct their own evaluations as distinct from an external team of evaluators, both formative and summative variations of evaluation can be used together in some form of inter-relationship. In this situation the distinction between the two is usually of degree of relationship. Formative evaluation is used as a progressive and continuous element with early feed-back that guides and influences the actual shaping of the curriculum through a series of successive revisions. Summative evaluation focuses mainly on the emergent curriculum and is end-on at the end of significant parts of it such as a 'term', 'unit', 'module', or 'year', or conclusion of a distinctive course. The inter-relationship of the two forms is necessary in the monitoring, control, and development of the nursing curriculum. Formative evaluation can be schematically represented in a horizontal dimension (see Figure 6), and summative evaluation can be viewed in a vertical dimension (see Figure 7).

Figure 6: The horizontal dimension of formative evaluation

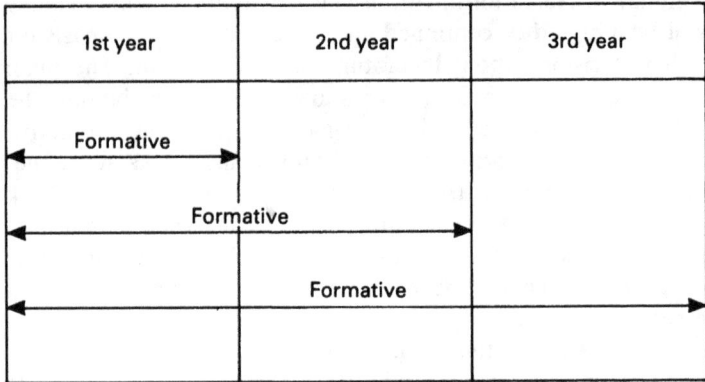

1st year	2nd year	3rd year
Formative		
Formative		
Formative		

Figure 7: The vertical dimension of summative evaluation

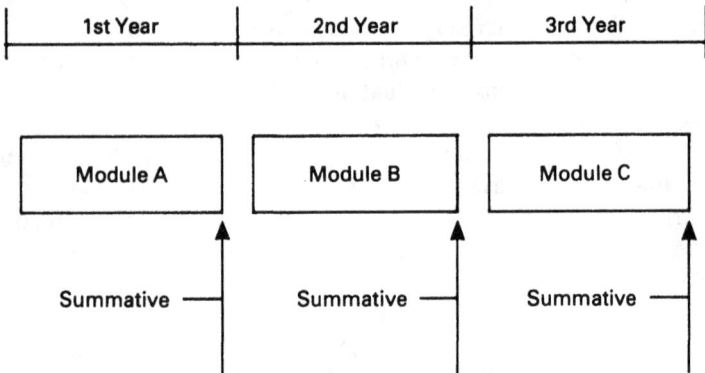

1st Year	2nd Year	3rd Year

Module A	Module B	Module C

Summative ⊣   Summative ⊣   Summative ⊣

SOME GENERAL PERSPECTIVES AND MODELS OF EVALUATION

Early models of evaluation were generally concerned with quality control and emphasised the need for feed-back to improve courses. Cronbach (1963) stressed the need to identify aspects of the course where revision was seen as desirable. Baker and Alkin (1973) focused on evaluation as being an integral part of course development itself in the formative sense. Smith (1965) described the central purpose as one of quality control and course improvement. Course developers sought two types of feed-back, testing the ability of students to carry out skills and procedures learned, and identifying discrepancies between student performance on the course and the ability to transfer these to the occupational roles on the job. This particular focus was very much concerned with the 'relevancy factor' of whether knowledge and skills learned could be effectively transferred as theory to practice in the working situation in which students would later find themselves. Clearly with nursing courses this factor of transfer and relevance is important, particularly with a nursing curriculum which is hospital-based and students seen to be a central part of the nursing work force.

Later models of evaluation have tended to take a broader perspective though each developed a distinctive set of educational evaluation characteristics. Stake (1967), Scriven (1973), Stufflebeam *et al.* (1971), Sanders and Cunningham (1973), Rippey (1973), developed models which are general enough to be applied to educational evaluation in a wide range of differing contexts. Stake (1967) was very much concerned with the response between the intentions of the curriculum and the degree of congruence with the actual outcomes through observation. In this model it is essential that the evaluators are external and the approach is summative and was thought to have an independence and objectivity that could not be achieved by internal evaluators. Scriven (1973) also placed value on the external approach and feels that evaluation is best carried out by people other than those responsible for the design and implementation of the curriculum. This approach became known as the 'goal free' evaluation which calls for the summative evaluator to assess the actual effects of the course and according to Scriven, should be done without knowledge of the designers' purposes, goals, or objectives of the programme.

Traditional external evaluations carried out by representatives of the statutory nursing bodies have in the past taken approaches more in line with Stake's model, although they have also taken account of the more formative evaluation evidence of the internal evaluators as well. A collaborative approach now seems to be very much developing within which external and internal evidence is shared and used to make final decisions and judgements. This approach is sometimes referred to as 'validation in partnership'. Stufflebeam and his collaborators (1971) place much less emphasis on the external evaluators and focus on the need to make evaluation data available for immediate decision making through the use of formative internal approaches. The direct concern is with the provision of continuous feed-back particularly during curriculum implementation and ultimately the successive re-cycling of its courses. The vital concern is with making successive improvements to courses and the necessary adjustments to keep intentions and outcomes in line and to measure the quality and effectiveness of the course in action. It seems logical that both internal and external evaluations have a significant part to play in the evaluation of nursing curriculum, and that eclectic use needs to be made of the different elements of the existing evaluation models. To be effective evaluation must be a co-operative effort and for valid and useful conclusions to be reached it is essential to achieve agreement between the evaluators concerned whether they be internal or external.

Two further evaluation approaches are worthy of consideration and both tend to take a more generic application to judging the effectiveness of a curriculum. They are respectively 'transactional' evaluation, and 'illuminative' evaluation, both are concerned with the importance of the perceptions of a wide range of participants in the curriculum including the course developers and the course users. Transactional evaluation Rippey (1973), and Seidel (1975), focuses on the effects of the perceptions of the design team members and the curriculum users. It seeks to give an 'instant' picture of what is happening in a curriculum at any one time and a collection of these 'instant' views provides a general over-view or complete picture of the situation. The methods used try to obtain data from opinions of the participants with opinions often acquired through active discussion. The concern is to provide information about where a course is at a particular point in time and to decide the direction in which the participants want it to move in the future. It attempts to identify and present problems in the course and also seeks to clarify the understanding of goals and possible solutions to perceived problems.

Illuminative evaluation characterised by Parlett and Hamilton (1972) attempts to 'illuminate' or throw light on the curriculum. They see transactions as a series of countless encounters of students with teachers, students with students and teachers with teachers, paying attention to interpersonal relationships, the use of in-depth interviewing and the use of a wide range of 'anthropological' methods to secure information and opinion. The anthropological methods include approaches such as participant observation, structured and non-structured interviews, questionnaires, written responses, recorded oral responses, interviews with individuals, interviews with groups, reports by course members, teachers and managers, check lists, documents, minutes of meetings and the like. Often a triangulation approach is used to gather accounts of the teacher–learner situation from three points of view, those of teacher, learner, and participant observer, using multiple methods to study the same activity.

GENERAL APPROACHES TO EVALUATION

Evaluation can be formal or informal or a combination of both. The formal approach tends to be rather rigid and seeks a high level of credibility and validity. The informal approach is more flexible and subjective and tries to throw light on the working of the curriculum as a whole. The best known approaches to evaluation can be classified generally as follows:

Case particular. Focused on an individual course or a major course unit.

Generalisation approach. Takes a very broad overall approach and concentrates for instance on the whole of nurse education in the United Kingdom.

Product evaluation. Focused on the product or outcomes from the course; for nursing these may be viewed as the occupational, professional, and educational pay-offs.

Process evaluation. This is concerned with the means by which the ends are achieved and is often directed towards the educational means and values, including the way in which the learning and content are viewed as a set of processes. The priority here is the intrinsic value of the educational experience itself.

Pre-ordinate. This is oriented towards goals, objectives, hypotheses, and anticipated outcomes. There is much concern in this approach with scientific measurement and quantification and the 'numbers game' dominates investigation

Holistic. A holistic perspective is taken and everything is considered or taken into account. Evaluation takes a rather wide-angled focus on things in general.

Analytic. This is directly the opposite to the holistic approach and looks at quite specific aspects of a number of elements by a method known as factor analysis.

Internal. Done by people on the inside and tends to be more formative but can involve summative approaches.

External. This is done by people from the outside who may have no vested interest in the course other than concern for quality and academic and professional standards. The usual approach is summative but collaboration on formative internal findings may take place.

The degree of formality or informality varies with each approach and is influenced by the extent to which evaluators are free to raise issues, interpret findings and advise or negotiate changes to be made. It is clear with most evaluations that judgement is a central concern with the evaluators and there is little real evidence to date to suggest that any one method of evaluating has significant comprehensive advantage over the others. There are good and bad elements in each form of approach and there needs to be an eclectic choice as far as these recognised methods are concerned, using moderate approaches rather than any one radical dogmatic approach.

The traditional approach in general and nursing education in the more recent past has been very much towards what has become known as 'the agricultural–botany paradigm'. Proponents of this approach have been Bloom (1970), Tyler (1950), and Popham (1975). In direct opposition to this have been the proponents of the 'illuminative paradigm' with significant support from Stenhouse (1975), Parlett and Hamilton (1972), MacDonald (1970), Jackson (1968), and Young (1971). Stake (1967) appears to take a moderate line operating somewhere between the two paradigms. It would seem that the moderate approach has most to offer for the evaluation of nursing education but an analysis of the two paradigms would be useful at this point.

The agricultural-botany paradigm

This approach is derived from experimental and mental testing schools seen in psychology and the significant feature is measurement or psychometrics. The method focuses on testing and scientific measurement. Objectives, the end product, achievement of pre-specified criteria are the standard concern of the evaluators. The students are treated rather like 'plants' and are given pre-tests (seedlings are weighed and measured) and submitted to different experiences (treatments and conditions). Subsequently after a suitable period of time their attainment (growth or yield) is measured to indicate the relative efficiency of the methods (fertilisers) used. The evaluations are designed to yield data which is objective, numerical, and which permits statistical analysis. Isolated variables such as IQ, social class, test scores, personality profiles and attitude ratings are codified and processed to indicate the efficiency of the new curriculum and its materials and methods. This form of evaluation, it is argued by its opponents, is based purely on the quantitative measurement of numbers and hence is viewed as a 'numbers game'. Such hard-line measurement of goal achievement can never be unequivocal and to rely totally on this form of evaluation as a utopian approach is counter-productive in educational assessment.

The sociological-anthropological paradigm

This approach is rooted in sociological and anthropological methodology and seeks to describe and interpret rather than measure. It sets out to take account of the various contexts in which educational innovations function. The central concern here is with the teaching and learning environment and the learning milieu with the focus on the operational curriculum, its emerging issues and related decision making. The techniques used are based on criticism, portrayal, and case study, and the aim is to study innovative projects and how they work. The evaluators seek to address and to 'illuminate' a complex array of issues that relate to the quality of the curriculum, hence the qualitative methods are emphasised. It does not try to use the standardised evaluation packages but aims to be adaptable and eclectic and the problems define the methods used not vice-versa. Problems are often viewed from several angles (the triangulation approach), and no method is used in isolation. The name of the game is observation, inquiring further and seeking to explain and unravel the significant features and to delineate cycles of cause and effect. The central method is participant observation and the production of continuous on-going records of events to organise the data at its source. Teachers, students, and other significant observers form a triangulation of evaluation relationships through the use of recorded discussions, interviews and questionnaires. The participants' written comments with documentary background information, committee minutes, autobiographical and eye witness accounts, recordings of meetings, and student assignments form the type of data used. The concentration is on information and data gathering rather than initially on decision making, and the priority task is to provide a comprehensive understanding of the complex reality of the curriculum in action and to illuminate its effects.

This overall approach does have critics who argue that it is too subjective, rather impressionistic, and without objective truth. It is important to see that the qualitative approaches consistent with the illuminative school do not reject outright the quantitative methods of the measurement school, but they do reject the assumption that objectivity can only be obtained through traditional quantitative scientific method.

QUALITATIVE METHODS AND THE NURSING CURRICULUM

The use of the qualitative evaluation approaches as characterised in the illuminative school may well enable a more complete and comprehensive evaluation picture of the nursing curriculum to be achieved, rather than relying too heavily on the usual conventional methods used in the past.

Because qualitative methods tend to focus on the processes of the curriculum rather than just its outcomes they are much more likely to identify the causes of success and failure. Clearly efforts in the past to evaluate nursing educational practices have to a greater extent failed to adequately serve the needs of those who require evidence of the effects of such practices. What then is the position for the nursing curriculum with regard to the two opposing paradigms? Nursing has been firmly entrenched in the psychometric tradition of the measurement school, at least for the evaluation of student performance. To what extent can the socio-anthropological methodology be used in the evaluation of the nursing curriculum? The illuminative evaluatory methods outlined above could be legitimately used to focus on the evaluation of students, teachers, the general operation of the courses, the functioning of the schools of nursing and their clinical experience areas in the hospitals and the community. Bendall (1971) has demonstrated sufficiently well enough that there is little positive relationship between theory and practice in the preparation of nurses for their roles in clinical nursing practice. This limited relationship is significant for any evaluation process in a curriculum where measurement of learning concerning nursing knowledge and skills is of central importance. It is well known that the present students of nursing are caught firmly between the diametrically opposed influences of school theory and hospital practice. It now exists to such an extent that students are continuously faced with serious inconsistencies in theory and practice. This inconsistency is maintained because both nurse educators and nurse practitioners hold logically incongruent views about the realities of nursing which produce major evaluation problems relating to the quality of skills and knowledge they are trying to learn. Nurse educationalists and practitioners must be brought closer together in the evaluation of the curriculum to help resolve some of their differences and to develop a shared responsibility for monitoring future curricula. This is more likely to happen if increased use is made of the more flexible approaches of the socio-anthropological paradigm.

The current trend of using curriculum development and evaluation groups at local level will do much to improve the relationships and to resolve differences between the nurse educators and nurse practitioners. This form of contact group could fall very nicely into the range and nature of methodology which is consistent with qualitative evaluation. The present shift towards continuous assessment methods is laudable and shows that nurse education is trying to move from a traditional hard-line testing approach to more culminative procedures that give emphasis to feed-back and provision of on-going knowledge of results. Normative, standardised, and criteria-referenced testing will for the moment no doubt continue as part of the overall methodology, but there is a pressing need to develop a much wider range of information-gathering techniques and to make more effective use of the information obtained about student learning experiences. Students' opinions and their self perceptions are important for evaluation purposes, particularly in relationship to their performance and ability to apply theory to practice. From an evaluation point of view new thinking is required to produce creative ways to test conceptual development in students and to diagnose learning difficulties. It is through the use of observational methodology that improvement can be made to gain first hand information of student ability in problem-solving situations, seeking information and evidence, looking at the nature of evidence, interpreting and analysing information and testing the practical application of theory in a variety of practical nursing contexts.

An illuminative approach to evaluation could be a significant step towards a quality focus in the nursing curriculum. Amongst the wide range of areas that might be investigated are the effects of curriculum implementation, the effects of teaching and learning styles used, the achievement of goals and objectives, the attitudes and relationships between educators and practitioners, the effects of examinations and assessment procedures, the allocation and utilisation of resources, and the effects of staff development and training. These examples are not exhaustive or in fact exclusive but rather an indication of the possible areas of concern. The interpretive character of the qualitative approach would allow a relatively in depth study of the nursing curriculum in action and at the same time elicit a wider data base. The evaluations would help to create a more coherent picture about the quality and effectiveness of the curriculum. The following general guidelines for curriculum evaluation in nursing education are offered:

Intentions and purposes

(1) Are the intentions and purposes, including a general

outline philosophy of the curriculum, clearly and concisely stated, and do they have central significance for the occupational and professional preparation of the nurse?

(2) Is the need for the particular course convincingly presented with appropriate supporting evidence and a rational justification for its development?

(3) Are all the major goals, general objectives and intended outcomes clearly identified?

(4) Are any potential difficulties and objections to the course anticipated, and are supporting arguments sufficiently valid, sound and rigorous to defend the curriculum?

(5) Does the course philosophy indicate in broad terms how the students will be changed by the course with respect to individual and personal development, educational and professional development?

(6) Is the type and importance of each major objective specified and is each objective relevant to the central aims?

(7) Are all the objectives precise, feasible, appropriate and achievable?

(8) If the objectives are achieved would the aims be realised?

Content of the course

(1) Does the content take clear account of the needs of the students as potential nursing practitioners and future professional nurses?

(2) Is the content relevant for them to meet and develop the appropriate professional and occupational roles that will be required of them?

(3) Does the content of the nursing curriculum have educational value, occupational utility and professional credibility?

(4) Is the content worthy of being included in a curriculum concerned with the preparation of nurses and will the material significantly help the student to be a good nurse, or the existing nurse to be a better nurse?

(5) Is the knowledge base of the curriculum clearly identified with appropriate eclectic use made of subjects that are necessary to under-pin nursing theory and practice?

(6) Are the eclectically-derived subjects sufficiently integrated into nursing practice applications?

(7) Is the specific 'nursing knowledge' clearly identified in terms of its central conceptual frameworks, conceptual nursing models, emerging theory, and current evolving practices?

(8) Are the broad range of nursing skills it is necessary for nurses to acquire included and are they sufficiently differentiated into their distinctive elements i.e. psycho-motor, cognitive, affective, communicative and interpersonal, behavioural, social, and technical?

(9) Does the content include major integrating and organisational themes, (the nursing process, health care maintenance, patient self-care teaching, holistic approaches) which can be used for focusing eclectic material into nursing contexts?

(10) Does the content selected allow the development in the students of attitudes, values and beliefs that the nursing profession holds in esteem and wishes to develop in its future practitioners?

(11) Does the common-core curriculum focus on nursing as its dominant concern and an application to practice?

(12) Is the content adequately sequenced and does it have progressive continuity and logical development?

Methods used on the course

(1) In linking methods to content, have appropriate choices been made with regard to themes, sub-themes, units and modules?

(2) Are learning and teaching methods clearly identified and incorporated as potential learning experiences?

(3) Is there a sufficient variety of teaching–learning experiences to meet individual student differences?

(4) Are the methods selected seeking to bring theory and practice closer together?

(5) Does the methodology to be used support an adult learning environment?

(6) Is there an appropriate balance of individualised, collaborative, and group approaches to learning?

(7) Is the teacher's role of facilitator of learning sufficiently identified and incorporated into the curriculum?

(8) Are there sufficiently clear and understood mechanisms operating which will allow the transfer of teaching and learning

into clinical settings in the hospital and the community?

(9) Have appropriate curriculum materials been developed or acquired in the form of text books, work books, study guides, ward learning profiles, advanced organisers, learning packages, computer assisted learning materials, and teaching–learning resources and technology?

(10) Do the methods used allow for the professional training of the student and the provision of an educational experience?

Course context

(1) Is the social and community context described in terms of local health provision and services which have relevance for the students in terms of the professional roles they would eventually play within these services?

(2) Is the institutional context in which the curriculum will operate explicit? This includes the school of nursing and the areas of experience that students will find themselves in for learning, working, and socialising.

(3) Is it clear how the curriculum fits, dovetails, or overlaps into the local environment whether it be hospital, local community, or other educational establishments and health care institutions?

(4) Are the lines of authority clear and understood by those involved and are there any other kinds of institution identified that could be involved or use the curriculum?

(5) Is the likely impact on other courses in the school of nursing or other institutions identified and are there any significant effects for teacher and resource allocations?

Assessment and examination of students

(1) Is the attainment of each objective evaluated by an explicit performance criterion?

(2) Are performance criteria congruent, complete, objective, reliable and efficient?

(3) Is the grading system clear and explicit and do grades reflect the priority among objectives?

(4) Do the gradings used ensure that critical objectives are achieved before pass or credits are awarded?

(5) To what extent is the evaluation of student performance based on formative or summative procedures?

(6) What is the precise nature of the overall assessment and examination component of the curriculum and how are distinctive student profiles determined?

(7) Is there evidence to suggest that students are over-assessed or under-assessed?

(8) Are the assessments sufficiently well distributed over the span of the course and is there a fair sampling of student ability over a wide range of course subjects and required skills?

(9) Are there available means of redress and appeal for the students with respect to conduct of their assessments and examinations and results reflecting referral or failure?

(10) What is the structure, function, and mode of operation of the examination board or committee?

Course logistics

(1) Are minimum and maximum numbers of students and intakes indicated?

(2) Are intakes recurring and are there any contingency plans for overload or shortfall of students?

(3) Are programme timings and experience allocations realistically calculated?

(4) Has the course been analysed for cost effectiveness?

(5) Are all the specified resources realistic and available for the course?

(6) Is there a planned strategy and realistic timetable for the implementation of the curriculum and are roles and responsibilities clearly defined?

CONCLUSIONS

The above criteria indicate the wide range of evaluatory activities necessary in order to secure appropriate information and ultimately make valid and reliable judgements about the nursing curriculum. By the end of an evaluation the curriculum should have been challenged, analysed, tested, and corrected, yet at the same time left intact as an educational system, but significantly improved upon. The objective is not to destroy the curriculum through critical analysis, but to influence its improvement and development in the most equitable way possible.

7

Implementation of the Curriculum: Innovation and Change in Nursing Education

Nursing education in the United Kingdom is on the threshold of a period of profound change following the publication of three significant reports. These are respectively, the Royal College of Nursing's Commission Report (Judge, 1985), the English National Board's consultation document (1985), and the United Kingdom Central Council's Project 2000 (1986). The response of the nursing profession to the proposals in these documents will to a great extent determine the nature of the occupational and professional preparation of nurses for several decades to come. The nature and direction of nursing education will as a result undergo far reaching change, both curricular and organisational, in response to the innovative effects that have their antecedents in the educational thinking of these committees. The extent to which the resulting innovations are effectively implemented will depend on the profession's reaction to them and its ability to cope with the change mechanisms involved.

Traditional practices and assumptions will be challenged, social and organisational relationships placed under stress, and operational roles brought into question. The success or lack of success in the implementation of the resulting new curriculum will depend on the extent to which nurse educators and others involved can develop the correct change-related values and competencies and a clear perception of the characteristics of the innovation and its effects upon the educational and organisational climate. The degree of tolerance and supportiveness, the extent of functional flexibility and openness to new ideas, and the motivational climate within which the changes will take place, will be the key factors affecting the implementation of the new curriculum. It will be necessary to identify a strategy for curricular innovation and implementation in order to facilitate a smooth change from the old to the new educational system. A critical need will be to discover the extent of positive and negative response to the new thinking and to point up the potential problem areas in relationship to likely 'change reactions' resulting from attempts to implement the new curriculum.

CURRICULUM INNOVATION AND CHANGE

The classical form of the stages of innovation suggest a logical sequence of initiation, development, dissemination and implementation. Several studies have shown that this approach is transcended by a very wide range of context variables which if ignored may well cause the most carefully designed and developed curriculum to flounder. The literature reveals that a large number of writers have stressed the need to take account of the environment in which the implementation of an innovation will take place. They include Schon (1971) with the 'centre-periphery model', 'proliferation of centres model', and the 'periphery-centre model'. Havelock (1973) in his 'social interaction model' and in his 'problem solving model' is confronted by the fluid and dynamic nature of the environment in which the models are to operate. Studies on 'organisational climate' (Halpin and Croft, 1963; Shipham, 1972); on 'organisational health' (Miles, 1965); on 'group-conformity' (Blau and Scott, 1962); on 'supportive climate' (Fox and Lippett, 1964; Sieber, 1968), have investigated relationships between innovativeness and specific variables of which most of the evidence points toward attitude and conflict difficulties. Festinger (1964) discovered that change in attitude towards an innovation does not always lead to behavioural change, and in fact the overt behaviour of individuals in a formal organisational setting may be highly divergent from their attitudes and centrally held views. McGeown (1980, p147) has also found that 'innovativeness' comprises a number of dimensions which are significantly related to a school's original organisational climate for change, its openness to influence, its supportiveness and motivational climate and to the major innovation, decision-making behaviour.

In considering a number of studies related to the teacher's part in innovation McGeown conceptualises teacher innovativeness as a multi-dimensional construct, including teachers' attitudes towards the adoption of specific innovations, their general change-related values, their adoption of innovations, their internalisation of adopted innovations, and their continual participation in change related professional activities (McGeown, 1980, p147). His conclusions are that teachers' internalisation and implementation of innovations appear to have a much more complex and subtle set of correlates and determinants which may account for failures in the implementation of innovations which have been adopted. He argues for further investigations of teacher's change-related values, competencies, and perceptions of the innovation.

Attitudes to innovation in organisational contexts

In addition to the above studies, important contributions to the literature by Rogers (1962), and Rogers and Shoemaker (1971), on 'attitudes to innovation', and Pratt (1980) on 'antagonists to change' indicate important necessary considerations for both individual and group responses within the innovatory environment. Rogers puts forward the idea of a continuum of 'dispositions' towards innovations based on studies in education, agriculture, and medicine. Rogers (1962), Rogers and Shoemaker (1971), Pratt (1980, p427), adopted this model to curriculum innovation in the following way. 'Enthusiasts' are characterised by vigour and independence of outlook, need adventure, enjoy making changes and take risks. They are regarded as gregarious and are likely to have had contact with other change agents and sources of information. They are likely to participate in the design and testing of the innovation. 'Supporters' are seen as respected members of the organisation, usually have a less radical image than the enthusiasts, but like the enthusiasts, they are actively involved in professional associations. They are knowledgeable about curriculum issues and are quickly persuaded of the value of an innovation once it has been thoroughly planned, justified and tested. 'Acquiescers' deliberate in their approach to change, will consider change, but will not initiate it. They tend to take the line of least resistance and adopt change, at least superficially. 'Laggards' have a low profile within the organisation, have few outside contacts, are usually sceptical about change. They are fixed in their approaches, and do not change until the majority of their peers have done so. 'Antagonists' are loners and they resist change actively or passively, sabotaging innovations as they are proposed or introduced. Through these characteristics Pratt sees a perceptible relationship between personality type and attitude to change. Since individuals may shift categories, an enthusiast for one type of change may become an antagonist for another. Pratt therefore suggests that it is best to consider the model as suggesting a possible spectrum of reactions and a strategy for change must work along the continuum, recruiting the first four groups and at least disarming the 'antagonists'.

The attitudinal problem can be further traced to the work of Freud (1922), Dewey (1916) and Lewin (1948), and further established in the 'normative re-educative strategies' through Bennis, Benne and Chinn (1969). The underpinning assumption is that how the client understands his problem is of central importance to overcoming difficulties normally created through inflexibility and an unclear conceptualisation. The important implementation factor clearly appears to be not necessarily the new ideas themselves but rather a matter of changing people's existing attitudes, values and relationships, and the change in attitudes is therefore as significant as the materialistic changes themselves and perhaps more difficult to accomplish. This means taking account of the innovation implementor user's value systems and the success of the innovation may depend upon persuading significant people in the nursing educational environment to accept the innovation and to secure the motivation of those involved. It is essential that persons involved whether they be clinical practitioners, educational practitioners, or managers and administrators, develop a changing pattern of practice as they are brought to change their old patterns of working and develop commitment to the new ones.

Bennis et al. (1969) also suggest an 'empirical-rational' strategy through which there are appeals to man's rationality and optimism, in that, if the best ways are demonstrated and an innovation is clearly seen to be justified and effective and consultation is carried out, the organisation will respond positively to the proposed change. An alternative approach offered by Bennis and his collaborators is the 'power-coercive' strategy, a political administrative influence through which the imposition of power alters the conditions in which other people act by limiting alternatives or by shaping the consequences of their acts. Many educational systems (including nursing) are regulated and controlled by power-coercive factors, often legitimately backed. The statutory and professional bodies of nursing possess powers of control and influence, which if operated in particular ways can control and reshape the nursing educational system by effecting a specific process of change. The power of these controlling institutions is often held in the form of new information and policies and knowledge as potential power. The coercive and manipulative powers of these nursing bodies clearly can have profound and lasting influence on the re-shaping of nursing education and a redistribution of power and control. It is important that in the formulation and adoption of a new educational system all potential responses to the envisaged changes are identified and prepared for.

THE NATURE OF CHANGE AND THE NEW EDUCATIONAL SYSTEM

The parameters of change for nursing education over the next decade are important for the long-term development of the nursing profession. A parameter can be conceptualised as a constant or design characteristic of a system whose value determines the nature or behaviour of the system involved. Change parameters are in this sense seen to be characterised through rate, scale, degree, continuity and direction, and can be viewed as individual, collective, large-scale or small-scale change. The list of characteristics is not exhaustive (see Docking (1987) for useful change criteria). Taking account of the nature of the parameters will provide essential data from which it is more likely to secure the desired change behaviour necessary for implementation of the educational innovation. The nursing profession, which normally develops its changes in a conservative and incremental manner, is entering a period of potential rapid change away from the established traditional system of the occupational and professional preparation of its nurses. The period and nature of change involved will inevitably bring with it a risk of high instability and threat to the existing system. Changes in the role of the students and teachers, the nature of the curriculum, and the environment in which the curriculum operates, will be reflected in the current changes in social and health care needs in society and in a new educational focus in the schools of nursing. This new focus will transform the schools of nursing in response to these changing situations and requirements, which will mean that nurse educators and others involved in nursing education must innovate themselves and develop learning systems capable of developing the required transformation.

The scale of change will also have to be carefully monitored in relationship to the time of innovation adoption (acceptance of the new system and a commitment to its implementation), and implementation (the realisation of the intended new system). Failure to do so will produce a quite profound 'curricular lag' which is the development of a gap between the discussion and consultation stage of the changes and the extent to which schools adopt the changes and implement them successfully. The degree and extent of change also carry important implications for the new educational system and its curriculum. Whenever educational change in the past has been innovatorily inspired it has been necessary to know whether the shift of change has been superficial or fundamental in terms of its adoption. It has been clearly seen with attempts to implement the nursing process in the past, that a conceptual shift amongst nurse practitioners is required with commitment to the idea itself to bring about a fundamental change in practice. Without this commitment and the necessary changes in attitude to go with it the changes that occur are at the superficial level producing only 'lip-service' to the changes and no real change in the system. In other words superficial acceptance of the nursing process will not have a profound effect on nursing practice but a fundamental acceptance will produce a significant change. A fundamental acceptance of a new system depends to a greater extent on whether those who will be participating have a conceptual acceptance and meaningful understanding of the benefits and improvements involved, and that it is seen as a non-threatening situation to themselves.

NURSE EDUCATORS AND THE IMPLEMENTATION OF THE NEW EDUCATIONAL CURRICULUM

A most crucial requirement is that nurse educators and nurse educational managers should develop a clear conceptualisation of the curriculum changes involved and a strategy of implementation for the new educational innovation. A considerable amount of time will elapse between the stage of innovation and the stage of implementation, during which effective and clear communications are necessary for the dissemination of the innovation over the national network of nursing education institutions. At this stage the 'change agents' (the central controlling bodies) must remember that it is the practising nurse teachers, nurse practitioners and managers who will determine to a large extent whether or not an innovation is accepted in the fundamental sense. A priority for curriculum designers is to develop a clear explanatory language which is free from non-essential jargon but sufficiently precise to give the same meaning to all potential users. The designers and change agents need to keep technical terminology to a necessary minimum so that the implementors and users do not react with accusations of 'jargon' and 'gobbledegook'. Terms must mean the same to all who are involved in the implementation, therefore a low-key approach, but one which ensures mutually agreed meaning, is necessary. Terms such as 'common-core curriculum' or 'common foundation' must mean the same thing for designers and for the users. Administrators and designers must also be sensitive to the fact that when teachers adopt an innovation the initial results may not be exactly those intended. The first time a new curriculum is run through it may be no more successful than the one it has replaced. Few curriculum innovations are right first time round because as teachers implement an innovation the innovation itself often undergoes change through the process of adaptation to the particular needs of teachers, learners, and individual schools of nursing, and the individual environments of learning in the competing *milieu* of nursing service and community demands.

The implementation of the new system will be greatly facilitated if the organisational and design stages have been carefully executed. This could well be carried out as selected pilot schemes with careful monitoring and built in checks to act as safeguards.

Explicitness will be a necessary concern for responsible implementation with a need to focus on personal contact with the curriculum users by establishing clear communications, adequate resources and above all the right attitudinal climate. Ruddock (1980) has found when investigating discrimination in innovations that teachers need to build up their confidence as innovators by being given opportunity to perceive the potential of an innovation and be encouraged to make active and critical response. She also highlights the need for students and teachers to be seen as partners in classroom transactions and stresses the need for greater attention to be given to the process of induction to the innovation for both teachers and learners.

Inevitably at the implementation stage with the new curriculum there is a need to heed the advice of Stenhouse (1975), that a curriculum without shortcomings has no prospect of improvements and has therefore been insufficiently ambitious. Stenhouse rationalises this in the sense that it should not necessarily be right but intelligent and penetrating and as such its dilemmas should be important dilemmas, its shortcomings reflect real and important difficulties. There will of course be shortcomings in the new educational system which will be reflected in the curriculum for nursing. These must be identified and intelligent solutions sought through effective evaluations, which need to be carried out during the implementation and the initial cycles of the new scheme as a reshaping exercise throughout.

IMPLEMENTING THE NEW EDUCATIONAL SYSTEM AND THE CURRICULUM

During the 1980s there has been an increasing focus developing on general social change as it effects matters of health care. This has brought about implications for nursing and a pressing need for a changing nursing curriculum. Logically, nursing is attempting to move with these changes to stand in closer relationship with the current modifications in health ideology and the social changes reflecting new health care expectancies. Within this relationship nursing education will have to fulfill better than it has been doing, its most basic task of preparing students of nursing to take on an increasing professional role. This means it has to respond more positively to changing patterns of health care and public expectations. The extent to which the adoption and implementation of the new educational system is effective in realising these changes will depend considerably on the nature of the decision making and the credibility of the decision-making process used to transform the curriculum as a paper exercise into an operational one, or a 'curriculum in action'.

A number of variables will be important considerations in relation to the type of decision-making and the way in which decisions most effectively allow a smooth implementation and maintain stability of the system as a whole. Directors of nurse education by virtue of their position will have three important working relationships with their staff. First, the authority relationship through which their decisions are legitimised, second, the power relationship through which satisfaction or dissatisfaction of staff members needs will occur, and third, the influence relationship over the staff which is a relationship of mutuality and reciprocality, or what Bolam (1975, p394) has termed professional colleagueship. The critical influence relationship is outside the hierarchical relationship of authority and power. Duncan (1973) sees this influence relationship as a very subtle one probably mediated much more through informal person to person inter-relationships outside of a power authority coerciveness, and more in line with decisions actualised through persuasion. Certainly there is much to be said for the assumption that if influence is to have any real effect there must be a mutual and reciprocal nature involved. Professional teacher satisfaction and potential for achievement will be key variables involved. Patchen (1970) has shown that participation and involvement in decision-making are central to achievement at the face edge of the job. The extent of satisfaction or dissatisfaction will have a profound influence on implementation effectiveness and the degree to which change can be accommodated within a reshaped nursing educational system.

One of the most often mentioned sources of dissatisfaction is put forward by Belasco and Alutto (1972) as the frustration of the expanding desires of various organisational members (particularly teachers) for participation in the organisational decision-making process. Patchen (1970), Likert (1961), and Bennis (1967), have found that much higher job satisfaction is associated with trust, increased productivity, and in general a more effective organisational climate. Kahn (1964) has also presented evidence which specifically indicates that satisfaction is inversely related to job tension. In view of the above evidence, when being implemented innovations are more likely to have a smoother transition into the organisational contexts of the educational institutions where such desirable outcomes as trust, low role-conflict, low job tension, and more positive attitudes to the organisation exist. Effective and carefully-monitored decision-making is more likely in this respect to create the right sort of organisational climate. This means that the perceived compatibility of the innovation with existing values and practices already in operation and preceding implementation, must be taken account of and identified before major decisions and decision-making procedures are laid down and allowed to become operational. Decisions will have to be concerned to a greater extent with changing and reshaping established practices and procedures. These will be necessary and central to the success of the operation, but the decision-making mechanisms must avoid creating a sense of threat and alienation among the nursing educational staff and others involved, if their support and commitment is to be secured.

As innovations such as the new nurse educational system require new skills, new attitudes and new value orientations it seems logical to suppose that changes will be required in nurses' roles and relationships, in and between the existing nursing school staff, *inter alia* with the clinical practitioners and managers in the clinical settings of the organisation. Coercion and power directives will not be the best way to achieve these. One has to take account of the thinking of Bennis *et al.* (1969), and elect for a 'normative re-educative' strategy which takes account of humanistic perspectives and the unpredictability associated with human behaviour. The decision-making reflecting changes may well have to start with the individuals concerned (ward sisters, nurse teachers, managers) and their individual attitudes to the new system, and not necessarily only with the working structure in which they operate. There is a danger that they will accept the *status quo* of their existing situations which would mean that at the clinical end of the job the innovation would only evoke minor adjustments to the new educational practices within the new framework that could be taken for granted. The basis for meaningful change will therefore rest on the degree of consensus reached between different interest groups in the system such as nurse educators, nurse practitioners, administrators and managers. This will only be achieved through a decision-making system that is grounded in a conceptual understanding of the new system, mutual trust, commitment and co-operation. Such a philosophy underlines the need to address the basic question of whether the new nursing educational system outlined in the recent nursing reports is to be simply a superficial rationalisation of the system or whether it is to be a fundamental shift away from the long-established apprenticeship tradition.

Three essential perspectives are required in order to positively direct the new system. (1) The need to develop an on-going dialogue and study into the phenomenon of change and its implications for nursing education and practice. (2) The need to develop debate and continuous consultation on the implementation of the new system and its resulting curriculum changes. (3) The need for nurse educators, practitioners and managers to re-examine their current attitudes and practices with regard to re-shaping expertise and the development of a preparedness to respond to a changing pattern of nursing requirements both clinically and educationally.

A carefully planned implementation strategy is an essential pre-requisite for a comprehensive operation of the new system, to provide an adequate working framework for the nurse educational institutions. The inescapable issues are those related to the nature and form of decision-making processes, the decisions taken, and the ability of the nursing profession to create and adapt to changes of its own making. The educational preparedness of the curriculum users, their understanding of the new system, and a flexibility in established attitudes will be the most important variables relating to the degree of success of the new enterprise.

CHANGING THE CURRICULUM

Changing the curriculum means making the curriculum different in some way, to give it a new position, course or direction. This often means alteration to its philosophy by way of its aims and objectives, reviewing the content included, revising its methods, and re-thinking its evaluatory procedures. The basis for any major curriculum change is significantly to improve the existing curriculum. Before any changes can be initiated, therefore, a complete analysis is required of the existing curriculum, to identify its strengths and weaknesses and areas of compatibility with the new ideology. This analysis is usually carried out using data acquired through the normal formative and summative evaluation procedures of the old curriculum. From this data the assessment of future needs can be made along with a determination of what needs to be changed, and the selection of possible solutions to problems and the means by which the necessary changes can be achieved. The following seven-stage approach is suggested as a set of guiding criteria:

Stage one. If a curriculum development and evaluation group does not exist, one should be formed to act as a co-ordinating group for implementing the planned curriculum changes.

Stage two. Appraise the existing nursing and educational practices which are representative of the currently operating curriculum. Study carefully the existing curriculum and identify its strengths and weaknesses by considering its overall intentions and purposes, including the basic values and beliefs which are currently part of the school's philosophy. Consider the extent to which the curriculum is offering an educational and training experience for the students. Determine carefully any explicit distinctions between training and educational practices and seek to identify necessary readjustments where there appears to be weak training inputs or weak educational inputs. Identify clearly and reconsider the potential end product of the course in terms of the type of practitioner being produced and whether the roles to be developed are consistent with the changing roles of future practising nurses. To what extent have roles been extended or expanded in line with current occupational and professional changes in nursing? The new curriculum must take account of these changes and address itself to the effects of these changes and adjust its focus accordingly.

Stage three. Make a detailed study of the existing curriculum content to see whether it is still relevant and appropriate to meet a knowledge base adequate for the changing role of the professional nurse. This will mean giving consideration to whether the skills, attitudes, and knowledge to be learned are still worthwhile and whether the present developing conceptual frameworks of nursing knowledge are sufficiently represented in the curriculum.

Stage four. Establish criteria for decisions about what needs to go into the curriculum and what needs to come out, and how the curriculum materials and methods might be changed. The core material, as distinct from the eclectic material, should have a distinctive and recognisably central position and represent as much of the established nursing concepts and frames of reference as possible, given the current state of development of nursing knowledge. The eclectic content should be as far as possible applied to the specific nursing content (Greaves, 1984), and should be used in such a way that it attempts to clarify, explain, and predict the current and future practices of nursing. Some attention will need to be given to the extent that the curriculum content is integrated to present a unified whole. This means reviewing the main themes and sub-themes in use and the possibility of introducing new themes that are more representative of current nursing values, beliefs, and practices. Similarly broad themes such as health and health maintenance, preventative nursing, communication and interpersonal skills, teaching and health education would be examples of realistic themes.

Equally as important as the subjects to be included is the way in which the content is dealt with to bring about the necessary learning in the students. A review of the teaching method, facilitation approaches and the way in which learning experiences are created for students is important. Is there sufficient link between theory and practice and are the current teaching–learning methods being used those that are most likely to bring about integration of theory and practice? While there is a need to increase the theoretical and intellectual demands within the curriculum such as logical thought and problem solving, there is also a need to locate the application of these to the practical realities of nursing care. This means to some extent considering the teaching and learning methods being used and determining whether there is sufficient variety of methods which will allow for both collaborative and independent approaches to learning. It also means deciding if the facilitatory function of the teacher is well enough developed to create 'learning' experiences for the students rather than operating entirely within a purely 'teaching' role. A review will also need to be carried out with respect to the current relevance of educational technology and curriculum materials. Such review would include appraisal of how well learning is packaged for students in terms of workbooks, study guides, advanced organisers, independent learning materials, computer-assisted learning, and distance learning packages. Many of these may need to be extended or rethought to fall in line with changed subject matter and new thinking in learning theory.

Stage five. This involves the design and writing of the new curriculum changes and these may include the revised philosophy and aims of the curriculum including the new intentions and purposes. It also includes the revised objectives and the reformed content and alterations to main themes and sub-themes along with any new teaching–learning approaches. Some of the existing evaluation procedures would need adjustments to fall in line with the new content and methodology.

Stage six. Within this stage the actual implementation of changes is put into action. Implementing the changes successfully involves having knowledge of the change environment and the securing of the participation of those people necessary to enable the implementation. Teachers, students, managers (both educational and clinical), and clinical nurse practitioners need to be involved and well informed with respect to the changes that are to take place. It may well mean for those involved the necessity to develop new competencies for modified or new roles, which would in themselves require further staff development training.

Stage seven. Following the implementation of the new changes it is important to evaluate the effects of those changes and it is with evaluation that this final stage is concerned. Evaluation is directed at the identification and collection of data and its analysis, in order for the effects of changes to be measured and appropriate decisions and judgements made.

The successful design and implementation of curriculum innovation and change is more likely to occur when a planned systematic strategy is adopted and a stage-by-stage sequence is recommended to achieve this. A sequenced procedure reduces the possibility of important things being overlooked and also focuses on the most significant elements of the curriculum. While a systematic approach involves a series of specific procedural steps, this should not imply that human judgement is abandoned during the implementation of curriculum innovation and change. On the contrary, those using a stage-by-stage approach must use it to organise and direct the thinking and planning required in the subsequent redesign of the curriculum by creating a focus within which the major change issues are dealt with.

Glossary of Terms

Aims. Broad statements of intention and purpose in the curriculum which usually precede the selection of content, methods, materials, and evaluation stages. Are often concerned with value judgements or major philosophical questions in the curriculum concerned. Act as indicators of direction in the curriculum and are used as guide lines rather than exact specifications. Frequently related to values of knowledge and understanding. Educational, professional, and occupational development of the student in the nursing curriculum. Nature of nursing and nursing education. Intentions and purposes of nursing, nursing education, and the school of nursing.

Autonomy. Freedom and responsibility over an area of professional practice i.e. the autonomy of the qualified nurse. Working within a discipline and using the rules to act autonomously with freedom to make decisions, based on the possession of specific skills and knowledge.

Behavioural objective. A learning objective which is pre-specified and leads to a relatively permanent change in the student's behaviour. Origins within behaviourist learning psychology. The behaviour of the student can be shaped and modified by the teacher and usually involves reinforcement. The concern is with what the student will be able to do at the end of the learning session involved. Behavioural objectives are extensively used in the nursing curriculum, usually following set criteria. Involves attempts to measure student performance.

Broad fields curriculum. An attempt to overcome the compartmentalisation of the curriculum by combining several subject areas into larger fields of knowledge i.e. 'combined studies'. It permits integration of subject matter and is an attempt to break down barriers between subjects.

Cognitive skills. Skills which involve thinking, knowing, comprehending, application, analysis and synthesis, which are dependent upon reasoned understanding and judgement.

119

Nursing activities are clearly dependent to a large extent on the practitioner's ability to analyse, reason, make decisions, and form judgements about nursing situations.

Concepts. Central and key concepts are essential in the curriculum as basic elements for developing meaning and understanding. To have a concept or idea helps to distinguish one thing from another and leads to a classification of the different aspects of nursing. Concepts in nursing education are essentially 'theoretical concepts' and are attempts to view nursing from a fairly wide angle to identify its nature and activities. The current development of conceptual nursing models are attempting to do this.

Conceptual frameworks. These are 'conceptual maps' used for mapping out the general structure of the curriculum. In the design of the curriculum conceptual frameworks are used to decide the general scope and level of content. With regard to the type of knowledge and skills to be included, they should integrate the key concepts concerned and indicate the disciplines to be included and the appropriate realms of meaning necessary for the study of nursing. Some models of nursing are presented as conceptual frameworks of nursing and are used in the curriculum to fit key concepts and basic themes required. The nursing process is often used as one of the central conceptual frames of reference in the curriculum.

Content. The knowledge, skills, attitudes and beliefs that will be taught, and which the students are to learn. It is the overall structure of knowledge and concerns that should, or should not be included. Considered as an essential stage in curriculum design and forms part of the rational curriculum plan. Involves decisions about selecting and choosing the appropriate disciplines, subjects and topics to be dealt with.

Continuity. Refers to the smooth linking of subjects and topics so that student learning can move smoothly from one area to the next. Related closely to other factors such as the scope and sequencing of content and the organising of learning experiences. Such links are sometimes called 'organising centres' in the curriculum. Based on the assumption that learning is a continuous process and each experience has an effect on the succeeding ones. The content and learning experiences should progress from one set of ideas to another set of ideas of increasing complexity. The experiences for the student should be presented in a sequence of subject matter which will lead to specific learning outcomes.

Core curriculum. Usually taken to mean the central area of concern, the central theme or thread which provides the 'main route' for the students through the curriculum or part of it. Can also mean the areas of the curriculum which are compulsory, rather than electives or special options. Some core curricular elements are distinctively based on specific learning approaches, such as problem-solving, or resource based learning.

Curriculum. Means much more than simply a course of study to be followed, and needs to be differentiated from 'syllabus' which is simply a list of subjects to be learned. Many definitions are available from general overviews to quite specific applications of the term. Kerr (1968, p16) calls it all the learning planned and guided by the school, whether carried out individually or in groups, inside or outside the school. Taba (1962) sees it as a rational planned design of educational activities which are calculated to diagnose needs, formulate objectives, select content, organise content, select learning experiences and organise learning experiences, and includes the evaluation of ways and means as part of the process. Stenhouse (1975) views it as an attempt to communicate the essential principles and features of an educational proposal in such a form that it is open to critical scrutiny and capable of effective translation into practice. A general definition could be the sum of learning activities and experiences that a student has under the auspices of the school. Clearly it includes intentions and purposes, content to be learned, methods of teaching and learning, The process of organisation, and the ways of evaluating its results and effectiveness.

Curriculum development. A planned systematic attempt to develop the curriculum. It involves the development of objectives, content, teaching and learning methods, the written curriculum materials and their testing, and their implementation

121

and dissemination through the school or college system. It also includes their quality control and evaluation. It may essentially involve in-service training for teachers for curriculum changes and the development of new skills to use innovatory methods and materials.

Curriculum materials. These are tangible resources used by the teacher and the students and include such things as study guides, workbooks, learning packages, and distance learning materials.

Curriculum methods. The teaching and learning techniques and ways of creating learning experiences for the students. Concerns all of the planned interaction between students and teachers, and includes the curriculum materials and resources to be used.

Curriculum process. Rational curriculum planning using a cyclical approach. Involves distinctive stages to determine and develop, objectives, selection of learning experiences, selection of content, the organisation of learning experiences and content, and evaluation approaches. Accredited to Wheeler (1967). Operates as a continuous and on-going activity.

Curriculum evaluation. See evaluation.

Disciplines. A discipline is a distinctive body of knowledge with its own rules, logic, and methods of scientific investigation. Disciplines have long-standing recognition and academic respectability. The major disciplines are part of the forms of knowledge which make up the traditional scholarly curriculum. Each discipline contains subject areas which in turn contain individual topics. The knowledge area of a discipline includes both its theories and practices. Nursing as yet has no distinctive body of knowledge in the true sense and the current development of nursing knowledge is only at the stage of conceptual identification and classification.

Eclectic. Selective borrowing of subject matter, usually from established disciplines. Certain elements are borrowed without necessarily accepting the values and beliefs of the total area of knowledge or range of methods involved in the discipline. The nursing curriculum eclectically uses knowledge from established disciplines (i.e. psychology, sociology, biology, anthropology) that helps the student to study nursing itself. Knowledge itself is not eclectic, but is eclectically used. The nursing curriculum uses material from existing disciplines in order to focus on the identification of a 'basis' for nursing knowledge and in this sense the knowledge serves as an antecedent to the development of nursing knowledge.

Epistemology. The study of knowledge is an important branch of philosophy which has important implications for the curriculum. What counts as knowledge in the nursing curriculum? Knowledge is usually seen as that which is believed to be 'true' and has some sort of acceptable evidence for that belief, either through experience or a recognised authority. The curriculum for nursing should seek to develop in the students understanding of knowledge based on evidence. What is nursing knowledge and what counts as evidence for claims in nursing theory and practice? According to Hirst (1969b) knowledge for the curriculum exists as 'forms of knowledge and understanding' and involves important decisions about what to include.

Evaluation. Concerned with attempts to judge the value, worth, quality, and effectiveness of the curriculum. Following the systematic collection of data and information, judgements and decisions are made in order to improve the curriculum in the light of the available evidence. It includes determining the extent to which intentions and purposes have been realised, and outcomes achieved. It also provides evidence regarding the learning achievements of the students and the degree of success of the planned learning experiences. Evaluation is similarly directed at the effectiveness of teacher performance, and the management and organisation of the curriculum. Evaluation may be summative (at the end of a course), or formative (continuous and ongoing), or combinations of both. There are many evaluation models available, which can be used within these two main formats of evaluation. Evaluation should meet various criteria, such as validity, consistency, reliability, although objective and subjective approaches both have parts to play. Evaluation should seek to improve the curriculum rather than simply point out its deficiencies.

123

Expressive objective. Developed by Eisner (1969) and differs from specific or behavioural objectives, in that an expressive objective does not specify the behaviour the student is to acquire after one or more learning experiences. It is described as an educational encounter or a situation in which the student is to work, or a problem with which they are to cope, or a task they are to learn. The outcome is not pre-specified.

Feed-back. Taken from cybernetics and systems theory. In the curriculum concerns built in loop-back procedures which provide information related to the assessment of students, and/or the monitoring of courses through established evaluation procedures. Feed-back to students, giving students knowledge of results of their performance in a specific piece of learning, or general progress. The effectiveness of feed-back is inversely related to its speed of operation within the system in order to correct faults and deal with shortcomings.

Formative evaluation. Evaluation which goes on during a course, rather than at the end of it. Provides information about aspects of the course where revision and correction is desirable, and provides evidence from which decisions can be taken to shape continuous improvement during the actual implementation and development of the curriculum.

Forms of knowledge. A philosophy of knowledge developed by Hirst (1969b), concerned with the need to make choices about the disciplines to be included in the curriculum. The forms of knowledge include formal logic and mathematics, the physical sciences, understanding our own and other's minds, moral judgements, aesthetic experience, religious belief, and philosophical understanding. Each has its own concepts, methods of enquiry and ways of establishing truth.

Fields of knowledge. Less specific than a discipline or form of knowledge, tends to include a number of subject areas (some of which may be taken from the traditional disciplines) where there is some commonality or relationship among the subjects, commonly related to an area of practice. Examples of fields of knowledge are 'educational studies', 'nursing studies', and 'management studies'.

Goals. Concerned with the intentions and purposes of the curriculum, and are usually found somewhere between aims and objectives. Some curriculum designers use goals as a form of 'general objective' or 'course objective' and in this respect are viewed as general statements of intent or directions to take in order to achieve the main aims of the course.

Hidden curriculum. What students learn in schools may be quite different from what they are intended to learn. As well as learning from the 'official curriculum' students learn a great deal by simply learning how to cope with the 'schooling' situation and the socialisation process with which they have to come to terms. In nursing education much of the students' reality learning in so-called planned clinical experience may vary considerably from the official planned curriculum. Again much of the hidden curriculum for student nurses is concerned with learning how to cope and how to come to terms with the system itself in order to learn that which is needed to survive the rites of passage through which they have to move during their training. See Treacy (1987) for a useful and extended account of nursing education.

Holistic curriculum. The curriculum addresses the sum total of all its learning experiences both in the school and beyond the institutional boundaries to wherever the learning is likely to take place. The range of influences considered are significantly wider and more profound. The curriculum for nursing students exists wherever the students are involved in learning whatever the contexts may be; hospital, community, patient's home, or the nursing school and its associated institutional settings.

Horizontal relationships. Those which run across the content of the curriculum, the loose horizontal 'links' between subject areas which seek to integrate different parts. Usually involve the development of agreed common objectives or learning experiences and is one way of developing the scope of the curriculum. Project work may be used to integrate a horizontal relationship between two or more subjects.

Independent learning. The learner decides his own course of action. Normally linked with learning rather than teaching and implies work done by the individual rather than in groups. In practice independent work is guided by the teacher or, at higher levels of learning, by a supervisor of some distinction (i.e. higher degree work), so in this sense there is collaboration. Individualised learning and independent learning are terms often confused in the curriculum, but they are not the same thing. While independent work is likely to be individual, individualised work is by no means necessarily independent, and may be strictly teacher-controlled.

Individualised learning. The planning and provision of individualised programmes of study, tailored to individual student needs based on the competencies and characteristics of the learners. Part of the reform movement today which seeks to introduce the individualisation of learning as a complementary method. Can be interpreted as simply providing tutorial assistance and guidance for students to facilitate independent study and the use of individualised learning materials.

Intentions and purposes. Address important philosophical considerations which are directed at the 'major' aims and objectives of the curriculum. Involve a series of value decisions about the nature of nursing and the professional and occupational preparation of nurses. What is the curriculum attempting to do, and how does it propose to do it? What are the reasons or justifications for the main aims?

Instruction. A North American term, the Anglicised meaning roughly means teaching and learning. The British use of the term instruction usually refers to a fairly narrow form of direct teaching with a skills orientation.

Instructional development. The planning done in direct support of student learning and the conditions under which it occurs. Includes the development of curriculum materials and the teaching and learning resources.

Integration. Breaking down barriers between subject areas and bringing essential areas of the curriculum together to form a unified and meaningful whole. The different subject areas should be considered in terms of their broad relationships and the extent to which they can be approximated for teaching and learning purposes. The integration should develop an organised curriculum which assists the student in securing, assimilating, and applying concepts and principles from appropriate disciplines, which can be applied to the study of nursing.

Interaction. Two forms of interaction are important in the nursing curriculum. The interaction between students and teachers which should result in the development of meaningful learning, the teacher–learner interaction. The second form of interaction is that which takes place between the nurse and the patient and is dependent on a range of skills which are central to the content of the curriculum.

Knowledge. A clear and certain mental perception which includes awareness, meaning, and understanding of something. Requires learning to achieve cognisance of facts and information in order to be understood. The possession of knowledge in this respect is to 'know' or to be aware and familiar with the possessed knowledge which has to be learned. Knowledge includes both theory and practice or 'knowing' and 'doing'. Distinctive knowledge includes related concepts, theories, principles, rules, axioms, methods of analysis, investigation and development. Intellectual and practical skills rest within the continuum of a knowledge area. In the nursing curriculum, knowledge of the established disciplines and of nursing itself should embrace the practice and performance of nursing.

Learning theory. There are many theories of learning, but there is no coherent theory which encompasses all aspects of learning. Learning is a complex activity and there are many different kinds. Some common forms of learning are mastering motor skills, memorising information, learning feelings and attitudes, concepts and intellectual skills, scientific inquiry and problem-solving.

Theoretical explanations seem to concentrate on certain types of learning or conditions under which learning is likely to take place. After reviewing many established theories of learning Hilgard (1956, pp486–7) developed the following propositions which are significant for curriculum design and development:

(1) In deciding who should learn what, the capacities of the learner are very important. Brighter people can learn things less

bright ones cannot learn; in general, older children can learn more rapidly than younger ones; the decline of ability with age, in adult years, depends upon what it is that is being learned.

(2) A motivated learner acquires what he learns more readily than one who is not motivated. The relevant motives include both general and specific ones, for example, desire to learn, need for achievement (general), desire for a certain reward or to avoid a threatened punishment (specific).

(3) Motivation that is too intense (especially pain, fear, anxiety) may be accompanied by distracting emotional states, so that excessive motivation may be less effective than moderate motivation for learning some kinds of tasks, especially those involving difficult discriminations.

(4) Learning under the control of reward is usually preferable to learning under the control of punishment. Correspondingly, learning motivated by success is preferable to learning motivated by failure. Even though the theoretical issue is still unresolved, the practical outcome must take into account the social by-products, which tend to be more favourable under reward than punishment.

(5) Learning under intrinsic motivation is preferable to learning under extrinsic motivation.

(6) Tolerance for failure is best taught through providing a backlog of success that compensates for experienced failure.

(7) Individuals need practise in setting realistic goals for themselves, goals neither so low as to elicit little effort nor so high as to foreordain failure. Realistic goal-setting leads to more satisfactory improvement than unrealistic goal setting.

(8) The personal history of the individual, his reaction to authority, for example, may hamper or enhance his ability to learn from the teacher.

(9) Active participation by a learner is preferable to passive reception when learning, for example from a lecture or a motion picture.

(10) Meaningful materials and meaningful tasks are learned more readily than nonsense materials and more readily than tasks not understood by the learner.

(11) There is no substitute for repetitive practice in the over-learning of skills (for instance, the performance of a concert pianist), or in the memorisation of unrelated facts that have to be automatised.

(12) Information about the nature of a good performance, knowledge of successful results, aid learning.

(13) Transfer to new tasks will be better if, in learning, the learner can discover relationships for himself, and if he has experience during learning of applying the principles within a variety of tasks.

(14) Spaced or distributed recalls are advantageous in fixing material that is to be long retained.

Learning experience. The participation by the student in a planned learning activity which enables some form of learning to take place. Learning experiences in the curriculum form part of the orthodox rational curriculum plan. They should be relevant, valid, comprehensive, and have pattern and variety of context. Experiences should provide the right conditions for meaningful learning, follow the correct logical and psychological sequence of learning, allow for necessary reinforcement, appropriate feedback and knowledge of the student's performance.

Model. Conceptually the word 'model' refers to a precise replication of something. It is also used to abstract an ideal such as a 'model nurse', or 'model society', or a 'model curriculum', in which case ideals are conceptualised in advance to demonstrate the feasibility and possibility that such an ideal might be a reality. A model can also be used to observe, order, clarify, and analyse structures, relationships and events. The process of model construction allows existing knowledge and events to be ordered and re-ordered, conceptualised and understood. For the curriculum, models can help to formulate intentions and purposes, identify priorities, select suitable content and materials, guide student and teacher interactions, evaluate effectiveness, clarify and implement educational arrangements, and guide development and change in the curriculum.

Modularised curriculum. The way in which the curriculum is broken down into units or parts for implementation at various levels in the school or school system.

Objectives. The intention of bringing about changes in the student's learning behaviour. An intention communicated by a statement proposing a prescribed change in a learner which

indicates what the behaviour is to be like when he has successfully completed the learning experience. See also intentions and
purposes.

Objectives model. Prescriptive curriculum model based on
clearly stated intentions and purposes, and indicating expected
learning outcomes and methods of achieving them. See Tyler
(1950), Taba (1962), Bloom (1956), Wheeler (1967), and Mager
(1962).

Organisation of the curriculum. An important stage in the
rational plan of the curriculum developed when the intentions,
content, and learning experiences have been decided. Intentions, content, and learning experiences are assembled and fitted
together in a logically integrated format.

Organising centres in the curriculum. The main frames of
reference or central focus of organisation, including the main
themes and sub-themes for the content of the curriculum,
sometimes organised as units, modules, or blocks of content.

Outcomes. Aims, goals and objectives which have been achieved
by the school by using inputs, processes and products. Part of a
systems approach to the curriculum.

Paradigm. A clearly established pattern of thinking developed as
a broad outline or framework of basic assumptions.

Parameter. In the curriculum it relates to the scale, dimension, or
general specifications of the curriculum, which usually include
the breadth and depth of treatment to be developed in the
planning of courses.

Problem-centred curriculum. The focus of the approach is to
problems which require contributions from a number of subject
areas to treat it adequately. Usually takes the form of an inter-
disciplinary enquiry.

Product. Refers to things developed along the way to achieving
the aims, goals, and objectives of the curriculum and might

include teaching and learning materials, curriculum packages and materials.

Process. Refers to those things which utilise inputs to the curriculum in order to meet the objectives and may include resources, particular methods of teaching and learning, the development and organisation of the learning climate. The term is also used with respect to the idea of a 'curriculum-process' in which objectives, content, methods, and evaluation form a rational approach to curriculum design and development.

Progression. A progressive approach of developing the curriculum in which a step-by-step method is used to proceed from the definition of ends to the development of the means to obtain the ends. Each step is retrocedal and self correcting. The term is also used to indicate a natural and logical development of sequence within topics and subjects that make up the content of the curriculum. A systematic progression through a subject.

Rational curriculum planning. A systematic method of curriculum planning, based on the objectives model and dealing with objectives, content, learning experiences, and evaluation, as a design and development sequence. Ideal for developing innovation and change in the curriculum.

Relevance. An essential criterion to be applied to the development of learning experiences. Often related to vocational needs in education. The curriculum for nursing should be relevant to the training, educational, and professional needs of the aspiring nurse.

Reliability. A criterion of evaluation for testing the curriculum for its quality and effectiveness.

Resources-based curriculum. A curriculum developed on resource-based learning ideas. The emphasis is on facilitating learning using a wide base of learning resources, often in a resource centre. Can take an integrated approach and leans on systems theory with frequent feed-back and knowledge of results for the students. Resources are viewed as teachers, technology, packages, distance learning modes, and developed curriculum materials. The teacher is viewed as an advisor, mentor, consultant, and facilitator for the student.

Scope. Refers to the horizontal relationships of sequence to the vertical in the integration of the curriculum. The term is also used to decide on criteria that will help in the selection of content and learning experiences. In this respect the word scope refers to the so called 'what criteria' and is central in considering what is to be included in the curriculum and this is sometimes referred to as 'determining the scope', or range of subject matter, and methodology to be used.

Sequence. Concerned with the vertical relationships in the curriculum and the systematic organisation of subjects in a suitable order for effective learning purposes. Follows the traditional learning criteria of known to unknown, simple to complex, concrete to abstract, increasing intellectual difficulty and the reiteration of central concepts. Closely related to scope in the integration of the curriculum. Sequence is closely concerned with the spatial relationships of content and processes and is sometimes referred to as the 'when criterion', or the point at which specific topics should be presented as learning experiences for the student.

Summative evaluation. This is the end-on type of evaluation and is concerned with the appraisal of the emergent curriculum. May be used at the end of a module, unit, term, year or completion of the course. It is usually used in conjunction with formative approaches, and both approaches are complemental rather than discrete.

Syllabus. A list of the content of a course or a collection of course topics which may or may not be in logical order.

Systems theory. Concerned with the study of complex entities. A system is an organised or complex whole or a combination of things or parts forming a complex or unified whole. Systems theory used in the curriculum is usually based on an objectives model approach to course design and planning and involves distinctive self-regulating control and feed-back mechanisms.

Systems analysis. A variety of different systems can be analysed and made amenable to planning by the use of a general theory. It seeks to understand how the system works preparatory to influencing or controlling it. Involves the identification of component parts and how they relate to or interact with each other.

Unity. Concerned with the idea of completeness or wholeness. The curriculum should have a distinctively balanced and integrated structure. The total unity may be brought about by the creation of many individual units of learning (modules as one example), where each one is a completed entity in itself, yet can be sequenced or related to other complementary units of learning.

Validity. A criterion of content, learning experiences and evaluation. Each should relate to the curriculum objectives. The content, learning experiences and evaluation approaches must be valid in order to achieve the desired outcome of the course.

Vertical relationships. The vertical linkage of sequence and continuity used in organising the structure of the curriculum and its organisation of content. Used in close and often overlapping proximity to the horizontal relationships to form an integrating matrix.

Bibliography

Baker, E. L. and Alkin, M. C. (1973) 'Formative evaluation of instructional development', *AV Communication Review*, Winter, pp. 389–418

Bandura, A. (1971) *Social Learning Theory*, New York, General Learning Press

Belasco, J. A. and Alutto, J. A. (1972) 'Decisional participation and teacher satisfaction', *Educational Administrative Quarterly*, Winter 1972, vol. 8, no. 1, pp. 44–58

Bendall, E. (1971) 'The learning process in student nurses: some problems and variables', *Nursing Times*, vol DX vii, pp. 43–4

Bennis, W. (1967) 'Beyond bureaucracy', in Hollander, E. P. and Hunt, R. G. (eds.) *Current Perspectives in Social Psychology*, Oxford University Press

Bennis, W., Benne, K. D. and Chinn, R. (eds.) (1969) *The Planning of Change*, New York, Rinehart and Winston (2nd edn)

Blau, P. M. and Scott, W. (1962) *Formal Organisations*, Chandler

Bloom, B. S. (1956) *Taxonomy of Educational Objectives, Volume 1, Cognitive Domain*, New York, McKay

Bloom, B. S., Krathwohl, D. and Masia, B. (1964) *Taxonomy of Educational Objectives, Book 11, Affective Domain*, New York, McKay

Bloom, B. S. (1970) 'Towards a theory of testing which includes measurement–evaluation–assessment' in Wittock, M. C. and Wiley, D. E., *The Evaluation of Instruction: Issues and Problems*, New York, Rinehart and Winston, pp. 25–50

Bobbitt, J. F. (1924) *How to Make a Curriculum*, Boston, Houghton Mifflin

Bolam, R. (1975) 'The management of educational change: towards a conceptual framework', in Houghton, V., McHugh, R. and Morgan, C. (eds.), *Management in Education. The Management of Organisations and Individuals*, Ward Lock Educational

Bruner, J. S. (1960) *The Process of Education*, New York, Vintage Books, Random House

Charter, W. W. and Waples, D. (1929) *The Commonwealth Teacher Training Study*, Chicago, University of Chicago Press

Colledge, M. M. and Jones, D. (1979) *Readings in Nursing. part two. Theoretical and Methodological Concepts of Nursing*, Edinburgh, Churchill Livingstone

Cronbach, L. J. (1963) 'Evaluation for course improvement,' *Teacher College Record*, Vol. 44, no. 8 pp. 672–83

Dale, E. (1967) 'Historical setting of programmed instruction' in Lange, P. (ed.), *Programmed Instruction*, Washington D. C., The National Society for the Study of Education

Dewey, J. (1916) *Democracy and Education*, New York, Macmillan

Dickinson, S. (1982) 'The nursing process and the professional status of nursing', Occasional paper vol. 78, no. 16, *Nursing Times*, vol. 78, no. 22

Docking, S. (1987) 'Curriculum innovation', in Allan, P. and Jolley, M. (eds.), *The Curriculum in Nursing Education*, London and Sydney, Croom Helm, pp. 149–63

Duncan, J. J. (1973) 'The Curriculum Director in curriculum change', *The Educational Forum*, vol. 38, no. 4, pp. 51–7

Eisner, E. W. (1967) 'Educational objectives: help or hindrance', *School Review*, vol. 75, pp. 250–60

Eisner, E. W. (1969) 'Instructional and expressive educational objectives: their formulation and use in the curriculum', in Popham, W. J., Eisner, E. W., Elliot, W., Sullivan, H. J. and Tyler, L. L., *Instructional Objectives*, American Educational Research Association Monograph Series on Curriculum Evaluation, no. 3, Chicago, Rand McNally

Festinger, L. (1964) 'Behavioural support for opinion change', *Public Opinion Quarterly*, vol. 28, pp. 404–18

Fox, R. S. and Lippitt, R. (1964) 'The innovation of classroom mental health practices', in Miles, M. (ed.), *Innovation in Education*, New York, Teachers' College Press, Columbia University

Freud, S. (1922) *Group Psychology and the Analysis of the Ego*, New York, International Psychoanalytic Press

Gagné, R. M. (1965) *The Conditions of Learning*, New York, Holt, Rinehart and Winston

Greaves, F. (1984) *Nurse Education and the Curriculum: a Curricular Model*, London and Sydney, Croom Helm

Grovenor, P. (1978) 'Nursing in theory' 1972–1977–1 *Nursing Times Occasional Paper*, vol. 74, no. 21

Halpin, A. W. and Croft, D. B. (1963) *Organisational Climate of Schools*, (Mid West Administrative Centre), University of Chicago

Hardley, I. and Lee, D. J. (1970) 'The alternative route – social change and opportunity in technical education', *Sociology*, vol. 4, pp. 23–50

Harrow, A. J. (1972) *A Taxonomy of the Psycho-motor Domain*, New York, McKay

Havelock, R. G. (1973) in collaboration with Guskin, A., Frohman, M., Havelock, M., Hill, M. and Huker, J., *Planning for Innovation through Discrimination and Utilisation of Knowledge*, 4th printing, Ann Arbor, Michigan, Centre for Research on Utilisation of Scientific Knowledge

Hilgard, E. R. (1956) *Theories of Learning*, 2nd edn, Appleton Century Crofts

Hirst, P. (1969a) 'The curriculum', *Western European Education*, vol. 1, no. 1, pp. 31–48

Hirst, P. (1969b) *Knowledge and the Curriculum*, London, Routledge & Kegan Paul

Jackson, P. W. (1968) *Life in the Classroom*, Holt, Rinehart and Winston

Jarvis, P. and Gibson, S. (1985) *The Teacher Practitioner in Nursing, Midwifery and Health Visiting*, London and Sydney, Croom Helm

Kahn, R. (1964) *Organisational Stress*, New York, Wiley

Kerr, J. (1968) *Changing the Curriculum*, London, University of London Press

Knowles, M. S. (1980) *The Modern Practice of Adult Education: from pedagogy to andragogy*, New York, Cambridge Adult Education Co.

Krathwohl, D. R. (1964) *Taxonomy of Educational Objectives. 11 Affective Domain*, London, Longman

Lawson, K. H. (1979) *Philosophical Concepts and Values in Adult Education*, Open University Press

Lewin, K. (1948) *Resolving Social Conflicts*, New York, Harper

Likert, R. (1961) *New Patterns in Management*, New York, McGraw Hill

MacDonald, B. (1970) *The Evaluation of the Humanities Curriculum Project: a Holistic Approach*, Norwich, Centre for Applied Research in Education, University of East Anglia

McFarlane, E. A. (1980) 'Nursing theory: the comparison of four theoretical proposals', *Journal of Advanced Nursing* vol. 5, pp. 3–19

McGeown, V. (1980) 'Dimensions of teacher innovations', *British Educational Research Journal*, vol. 6, no. 2., pp. 47–63

Mager, R. F. (1962) *Preparing Instructional Objectives*, Palo Alto: Fearon

Miles, M. B. (1965) 'Planned change and organisational health: figure and ground' in Charlton, R. O. (ed.), *Change Process in the Public Schools*, University of Oregon, Centre for Advanced Study of Educational Administration

Orem, D. E. (ed.), (1979) *Concept Formalization in Nursing Process and Product*, (2nd edn), New York, McGraw Hill

Parlett, M. and Hamilton, D. (1972) 'Evaluation as illumination: a new approach to the study of innovatory programmes', *Occasional Paper 9 Centre for Research in Educational Sciences*, University of Edinburgh

Patchen, M. (1970) *Participation, Achievement and Involvement on the Job*, Engelwood Cliffs, New Jersey, Prentice Hall

Popham, W. J. (1975) *Educational Evaluation*, Engelwood Cliffs, New Jersey, Prentice Hall

Pratt, D. (1980) *Curriculum Design and Development*, New York, London, Harcourt Brace Jovanovich

Quinn, F. M. (1980) *The Principles and Practice of Nurse Education*, London and Sydney, Croom Helm.

Reid, N. G. (1985) *Wards in Chancery? Nurse Training in the Clinical Area*, London, Royal College of Nursing

Riehl, J. P. and Roy, C. (1980) *Conceptual Models for Nursing 2nd Edn*, Engelwood Cliffs, New Jersey, Prentice Hall

Rippey, R. (ed.) (1973) *Studies in Transactional Evaluation*, Berkeley, California, McCutchen Publishing Corporation

Rogers, E. M. (1962) *Diffusion of Innovation*, New York, Free Press

Rogers, E. M. and Shoemaker, F. (1971) *Communication of Innovations*, New York, Free Press

Ruddock, J. (1980) 'Insights into the process of dissemination', *British*

Educational Research Journal, vol. 6, no. 2, pp. 139–46

Salvage, J. (1985) *The Politics of Nursing*, London, Heinemann

Sanders, J. R. and Cunningham, D. J. (1973) 'A structure for formative evaluation in product development', *Review of Educational Research*, vol. 43, pp. 217–36

Schon, D. A. (1971) *Beyond the Stable State*, Temple Smith

Scriven, M. (1967) 'The methodology of evaluation', in Worthen, B. and Sanders, J. (eds.), *Educational Evaluation: Theory and Practice*, Worthington, Ohio, Charles A. Jones, pp. 60–104

Scriven, M. (1973) 'Goal free evaluation', in House, E. R. (ed.), *School Evaluation: the Politics and Process*, Berkeley, California, McCutchen Publishing Corporation

Seidel, R. J. (1975) 'Transactional evaluation. A technique for coping with human problems', in *Instructional Technology for Government Planners*, Conference proceedings, Washington D.C.: Inter-Agency Advisory Group, U.S. Civil Service Commission

Shiphan, M. D. (1972) 'The role of the teacher in selective innovative schools in the United Kingdom', in (OECD), *The Changing Role of the Teacher and its Implications*, OECD, Paris

Sieber, S.D. (1968) 'Organisational influences on innovative roles', in Eidellt, and Kitchell, L. (eds.), *Knowledge Production and Utilisation*, University of Oregon

Smith, R. G. (1965) *Controlling the Quality of Training*, Technical Report, no. 65–6. Alexandria, VA, Human Resources Research Organisation

Stake, R. E. (1967) 'The countenance of educational evaluation', *Teachers' College Record*, vol. 68, no. 7, University of Illinois

Stenhouse, L. (1970) 'Some limitations of the use of objectives in curriculum research and planning', *Pedagogica Europea*, pp. 75–83

Stenhouse, L. (1975) *An Introduction to Curriculum Research and Development*, Heinemann, London

Stufflebeam, D. L., Foley, W. J., Gephart, W. J., Guba, E.G., Hammond, R. I., Merriman, H. O. and Provus, M. M. (1971) *Educational Evaluation and Decision Making*, PDK National Study Committee on Evaluation, F. E. Peacock, Itasca, Illinois, pp. 92–104

Taba, H. (1962) *Curriculum Development Theory and Practice*, Harcourt Brace Jovanovich

Treacy, M. P. (1987) 'Some aspects of the hidden curriculum', in Allen, P. and Tolley, M. (eds.), *The Curriculum in Nursing Education*, London and Sydney, Croom Helm, pp. 164–75

Tyler, R. W. (1950) *The Basic Principles of Curriculum and Instruction*, Chicago, University of Chicago Press

Welch, L. B. and Slagle, J. C. (1980) 'Does integrated content lead to integrated curriculum' *Journal of Nursing Education*, vol. 19, pp. 38–40

Wheeler, D. K. (1967) *Curriculum Process*, London, Unibooks, University of London Press

Young, M. F. D. (1971) *Knowledge and Control*, New York, Collier Macmillan

Reports

English National Board for Nursing, Midwifery and Health Visiting. (1985) *Consultation Document on Professional Education/Training Courses*, ENB, London

The Royal College of Nursing (1985) *Commission on Nursing, (Chairman Judge, H.) Nurse Education: A New Dispensation*, RCN, London

The United Kingdom Central Council for Nursing, Midwifery and Health Visiting (1986) *Project 2000: A New Preparation for Practice*, UKCC, London

Index

For Product Safety Concerns and Information please contact our EU
representative GPSR@taylorandfrancis.com
Taylor & Francis Verlag GmbH, Kaufingerstraße 24, 80331 München, Germany

.